Anatomy: A Pressing Concern in Exercise Physiology

(Commitment to Professionalism)

Authored by

Tommy Boone

Board Certified Exercise Physiologist, USA

Anatomy: A Pressing Concern in Exercise Physiology

Commitment to Professionalism

Author: Tommy Boone

eISBN (Online): 978-1-68108-469-5

ISBN (Print): 978-1-68108-470-1

First published in 2017.

Bentham Science Publishers Ltd.
Executive Suite Y - 2
PO Box 7917, Saif Zone
Sharjah, U.A.E.
Email: subscriptions@benthamscience.org

BENTHAM SCIENCE

CONTENTS

FOREWORD

In simple straightforward language, Dr. Boone has set forth important reasons for teaching anatomy in the exercise physiology curriculum. He believes that the students of exercise physiology cannot do their best in prescribing exercise medicine without an understanding of anatomy. This is especially true when it comes to flexibility training.

Anatomy: A Pressing Concern in Exercise Physiology presents the first-ever anatomical background to why there are good, useless, and dangerous flexibility exercises. Dr. Boone believes that without anatomy as part of the exercise physiology curriculum, exercise physiologists will continue to engage their clients and patients in useless and dangerous flexibility exercises. The result is a failure to increase their range of motion, a waste of time in achieving increased flexibility, and the possibility of damage to the muscles and joints. Such a practice is similar to prescribing exercise medicine without an understanding of exercise duration, frequency, intensity.

While it is possible that the students of exercise physiology can learn anatomy without hands-on dissection, it is not the desired approach. That is why Dr. Boone developed an Anatomy Laboratory with cadavers that were dissected by his students at Wake Forest University in Winston-Salem, NC, the University of Southern Mississippi in Hattiesburg, MS, and the College of St. Scholastica in Duluth, MN.

This book explains that we must close the door on yesterday's views of "what is exercise physiology" and keep it closed. We live today, not yesterday. We are healthcare professionals who prescribe exercise medicine to prevent and treat chronic diseases and disabilities. This book is a big step into the 21st century commitment to the professionalization of exercise physiology.

Frank B. Wyatt
Department of Athletic Training & Exercise Physiology
Midwestern State University
Wichita Falls, TX
U.S.A

PREFACE

For years the kinesiology course was the anatomy course in the health and physical education degree. Now, although students can still major in health and physical education, the title has changed in many academic institutions to exercise science, kinesiology, and numerous other degree titles. It is no secret that exercise physiology grew from this academic background of athletics and exercise in health and disease. Today, exercise physiology is increasingly recognized as the new 21st century healthcare profession. While exercise physiologists are educated to prescribe exercise medicine from a physiological perspective, there is the concern that they need an anatomy course to fully understand the depth and implications of flexibility training.

This ebook, ***Anatomy: A Pressing Concern in Exercise Physiology***, is the opportunity to promote the academic importance of anatomy as part of the professional development of exercise physiologists. It describes in detail the anatomical reasons for the good, useless, and dangerous flexibility exercises. Without question, academic exercise physiologists should teach anatomy to the undergraduate and post-graduate students, and the students should have the same opportunity as other healthcare students to study cadavers to grasp the significance of the musculoskeletal system. The hands-on laboratory opportunities will help the students of exercise physiology to safely prescribe exercise medicine and to work as a professional with athletes of diverse sports. This work should also encourage the support and recognition of the ASEP Board Certified Exercise Physiologists as healthcare professionals.

CONFLICT OF INTEREST

The author confirms that author has no conflict of interest to declare for this publication.

ACKNOWLEDGEMENTS

Declared none.

Tommy Boone
Board Certified Exercise Physiologist
USA

Anatomy: A Pressing Concern in Exercise Physiology

CHAPTER 1

The Anatomy Challenge

Abstract: Although there is an explosion of computer-based human anatomy material available to teach anatomy, cadaveric dissection by students and the integration of knowledge from textbooks and didactic lectures are still the most popular methods of teaching anatomy. The volume of time dedicated to teaching anatomy has steadily decreased over the past several decades. This has resulted in more college graduates with an inadequate understanding of anatomy. Do you want students of exercise physiology to be taught by qualified teachers? If the answer is "yes" -- then you must act now. Commitment to professionalism is imperative.

Keywords : Applied anatomy, Biochemistry, Biomechanics, Cadavers, Exercise physiologist, Kinesiology, Physiology, Visualization.

INTRODUCTION

For the purpose of clarification, the term anatomy is the study of the structure of the human body. For decades, it has been synonymous with the content of the traditional kinesiology course in the physical education major. In fact, for many years, kinesiology was always the academic course that the majority of the physical education majors looked forward to studying. They understood that anatomy was necessary to teach and coach physical activities and sports.

From a historical perspective, when the name of many physical education departments was changed to kinesiology, exercise science, and numerous other similar titles during the 1960s and 1970s, the kinesiology course remained as part of the curriculum. After all, there was then and still is today the belief that kinesiology is understood to mean the "science of movement". Anatomy, as an integral academic area of study, has been firmly established in health and physical education.

Tommy Boone

The students were led to believe that the science of movement was synonymous with the anatomy of movement (Box **1**). That is why the kinesiology (*i.e.*, applied anatomy) course had been an important part of the academic course work in kinesiology and related academic majors. Most recently, in the late 1980s and 1990s, the emphasis away from teaching anatomy is clearly a radical change that reflects the emphasis on exercise physiology research.

Box 1. What is meant by the term anatomy?

The word **anatomy** is derived from a Greek word meaning "to cut up". The word anatomize was more commonly used than the word dissect. Human anatomy as a science has always been about dissection of the human body; whereas, the science of physiology is concerned with the function of the human body. The dissection of cadavers has served as the basis of understanding the structure and function of the human body. Most of the terms that make up anatomy are of Greek or Latin derivation. The study of anatomy has had a powerful influence on medicine and the understanding of how to take care of the body. Athletics in particular is linked to many forms of art and the sense of excellence in human form and movement.

With increased emphasis on research at the doctorate level, little to no attention has been given to applied anatomy. This has resulted in a significant decrease in doctorate prepared exercise physiologists, kinesiologists, and physical educators who can teach anatomy. Also, it is clear that the emphasis on biomechanics, graded exercise testing and prescription, and sports nutrition has served to some degree to diminish the teaching of bodily structure. Yet, an understanding of the structure and internal workings of the body is critical to a rigorous science-oriented education.

Hence, even though it was accepted years ago that anatomy was essential to the students' education, the exposure to anatomy today has decreased to essentially being non-existent in many academic majors. This means the majority of the students at academic institutions throughout the United States are unable to describe the muscles of the shoulder region and how they are different from the hip region. The students' education is inadequate and, therefore, is likely to have an adverse effect on their interaction with clients and patients. Most graduate without being able to identify specific muscles in the human body or attachment sites, innervations, functions, and variations.

While sport biomechanical principles are important, it should be obvious that an understanding of anatomy even more is critical to the students' education. It is very likely that this view is understood by academic exercise physiologists without having to elaborate on it. However, given the emphasis on research while pursuing the doctorate degree, the majority of the graduates are either not interested or unprepared to teach anatomy. As a result, the students graduate from college without the ability to accurately apply anatomical concepts to the human body at rest, during exercise, and when correcting musculoskeletal disabilities. No doubt that is why Somerset Maugham wrote in his book, *On Human Bondage*, about a lecturer advising first-year medical students that, "You will have to learn many tedious things which you will forget the moment you have passed your final examination, but in anatomy it is better to have learned and lost than never to have learned at all."

A strong base of functional human anatomy is thought to serve as the foundation for all subsequent exercise physiology courses. That is why functional human anatomy is considered as a cornerstone for exercise physiology practice. Several decades ago no one would have thought about graduating students interested in fitness programs and/or sports training without a solid grasp of applied anatomy. In fact, it was believed to be so important that college teachers actually taught origins, insertions, and functions of all the major muscles. After all, anatomy is a discipline with its own language to describe structures of the body that, then allows for an increased understanding of the physiology of the body as well.

The Language of Anatomy

Only a small percent of the exercise physiology teachers know how to teach students the language of anatomy. This point is more complex than it sounds, especially since it is not the same as being well-informed. In many ways, it is an entirely new mental frame of reference. Understanding functional anatomy is not just about memorizing the facts about muscles. It is also about having the knowledge and understanding that allows for determining whether an anatomical comment or statement either makes sense or not.

Understandably, anatomy is complex. It requires intellectual effort and time to identify specific structures and relationships (Box **2**). But, unfortunately, the perception that learning anatomy is little more than memorization, which has kept has kept it a secondary subject. However, this thinking is wrong. It also misses the point of an important three-dimensional view of anatomy. Students are taught facts, but they must also learn the ability to describe the "why".

Box 2. The anatomy education.

An **anatomy education** is not only an essential part of the curriculum -- it also helps to further the development of professionalism for members of the healing professions.

As an example, students must be able to explain anatomically why the brachialis is a stronger elbow flexor than the biceps brachii muscle. Figuring out what makes one muscle stronger than another or how the different muscles work together to carry out a specific function across a joint among other competing ideas is critical to speaking the language of anatomy. Thus, the goal is not to learn just that the brachialis flexes the elbow (*i.e.,* what to think), but why the brachialis is the powerhouse of the elbow flexors (*i.e.,* how to think). The rationale for this thinking is as follows.

Anyone who is responsible for sports training programs may understand that both muscles flex the elbow joint. But, as a healthcare professional, the exercise physiologist should understand the functional significance of the brachialis as a one-joint muscle that inserts on the ulna that permits only one motion (*i.e.,* flexion) when it contracts. The biceps brachii muscle is a two-joint muscle that inserts on a forearm bone that allows for lateral rotation of the radius as well as flexion of the elbow joint. In other words, knowing the origin and insertion of a muscle defines its functional limits.

That is why it is the responsibility of the teacher to be very specific with the presentation of each skeletal muscle. After all, a muscle's shape (as defined by its origin and insertion) gives rise to its function and/or its purpose. To grasp this point, students should be encouraged to ask questions and to look for anatomical information that justifies and/or clarifies their thinking when considering the musculoskeletal differences (*e.g.,* as just presented with the brachialis and the biceps brachii).

Information that comes with visualization (*i.e.*, mentally creating a mental image) of muscles is as simple as accessing information about specific muscles and their relationships. The ability to create mental images is the key to understanding the language of anatomy. Literally speaking, it means "to see in your mind a mental image of a muscle or muscles" and, then, to play the image dynamics over and over again. It is the process of transforming anatomical information into a visual picture that enables the student to observe, make sense, and understand the context of a muscle and its relationship to other muscles.

Because of the interest in fitness and athletics, it is believed that exercise physiologists know anatomy and can apply it to human movement to help reduce injuries and improve performance (Box **3**). Do you think this is true today? The truth is that it is not true. Doctorate prepared exercise physiologists with a thorough knowledge of anatomy are a diminishing pool of individuals. As stated earlier, the majority of the academic exercise physiology and/or related academic programs do not teach anatomy. This is especially true at the doctorate level. So, turning to a doctorate exercise physiologist, perhaps, one who was just recently hired at the assistant professor level to teach anatomy and cadaver dissection (*i.e.,* if both were to exist in the curriculum) is rather foolish.

Box 3. The academic exercise physiologist as the anatomy teacher.

Ideally, the anatomy teacher in the exercise physiology major should be an exercise physiologist who uses anatomy in his or her practice. Understanding anatomy as well as developmental anomalies is especially important to successfully confronting amorphous clinical entities, particularly as they relate to the function of muscles.

But, unfortunately, it is not all that self-evident in exercise physiology that academic exercise physiologists do not know anatomy. Moreover, in addition to the failure to teach anatomy at the doctorate level, there is little talk about the importance of an applied anatomy class or the course simply no longer exists since it was dropped from the academic major years earlier.

Only a few academic exercise physiologists are actually prepared to visualize, that is, to "see" anatomy (Box **4**). Ironically, these are the facts and, strangely enough, it has become all too obvious at a time when the students' knowledge of anatomy is critical to the safety of clients and patients in exercise medicine programs. This means that the profession of exercise physiology should create with great urgency career opportunities for exercise physiologists with training in anatomy.

Box 4. Good anatomy teachers can visualize anatomy.

Visualization is significantly enhanced with the opportunity to study and/or dissect cadavers. Clearly, the use of cadavers is at the core of teaching anatomy since the Renaissance. Persaud, TVN (1984) *The Early History of Human Anatomy: From Antiquity to the Beginning of the Modern Area.* Thomas Books, Springfield, Massachusetts.

If exercise physiologists were to argue that they can teach anatomy as well as they teach other exercise physiology courses, it simply cannot be true. Defining the anatomical site of a muscle or related muscles to resolve a question about weight lifting, flexibility, or a developmental anomaly is important if the exercise physiologist is to accurately convey a sound knowledge of anatomical structures and functions. This can only be achieved by an extensive study of functional anatomy. For example, consider the following questions?

1. How many muscles produce shoulder flexion?
    - Answer: 1, 2, 3, 4, 5
2. How many muscles contribute to shoulder flexion as a functional part of a larger muscle?
    - Answer: 1, 2, 3, 4, 5
3. How many shoulder flexors do not original from the anterior perspective of the body?
    - Answer: 1, 2, 3, 4, 5
4. How many shoulder flexors cross more than one joint?
    - Answer: 1, 2, 3, 4, 5
5. How many nerves contribute to shoulder flexion?
    - Answer: 1, 2, 3, 4, 5
6. How many nerves that contribute to shoulder flexion innervate more than one muscle?
    - Answer: 1, 2, 3, 4, 5

7. How many nerves that contribute to shoulder flexion contribute to elbow flexion?
    - Answer: 1, 2, 3, 4, 5
8. How many muscles at the shoulder joint perform both abduction and adduction of the upper limb?
    - Answer: 1, 2, 3, 4, 5
9. How many shoulder flexors perform inward rotation of the arm?
    - Answer: 1, 2, 3, 4, 5
10. How many shoulder flexors have a functional part that performs shoulder extension?
    - Answer: 1, 2, 3, 4, 5

Questions: 1, 2, 3, 4, 5, 6, 7, 8, 9, 10

Answers: 5, 2, 1, 1, 4, 1, 1, 2, 4, 1

Although these are simple and straight forward questions, there is no way to answer the questions correctly without studying the anatomy of the shoulder muscles and nerves (Box **5**). Unfortunately, this problem is only going to get worse over time. This means the students' understanding of the science of health and human movement will not improve, which is ultimately a negative outcome. This thinking is inconsistent with the anticipated academic and professional qualifications and standards of exercise physiologists as healthcare professionals.

Box 5. Hands-on is very important.

> One learns by doing the thing; for though you think you know it, you have no certainty until you try.
>
> – Sophocles

Any thinking otherwise (such as from the strength and conditioning perspective) is unlikely to generate the right answers. Essential to this perspective, that is, confronting those who act as though they know anatomy when they do not is hugely problematic. They are often heard to say, "Get serious. Who really cares about anatomy?" Of course that kind of thinking is seriously missing the point. It is also self-defeating because a thorough knowledge of anatomy is imperative to the professional education of all healthcare practitioners.

There should be no resistance to the importance of teaching anatomy, even on the level as common as is biochemistry. The valued of anatomy is on the same order as the other content areas in exercise physiology (*e.g.,* ECG, biomechanics, and cardiovascular physiology to mention a few) and yet, it is more than obvious that almost every other subject is emphasized more than the teaching of anatomy.

It's all about Physiology

Contrary to popular opinion, not knowing anatomy at the same level as students and teachers are expected to know, for example, the enzymatic steps in glycolysis or the role of Kreb's cycle in making electrons available to the electron transport system (ETS) makes little sense. Similarly, expecting students to know that cytochrome A_3 is the final electron acceptor for molecular oxygen, thus allowing for the oxidative phosphorylation of ADP to ATP, while not expecting or even teaching students to know that the superior gluteal nerve innervates the tensor fascia latae, gluteus medius, and gluteus minimus make no sense much less not knowing why the muscles function as they do individually and/or collectively at the hip joint as primary abductors of the lower limb.

The academic exercise physiologist's interest in biochemistry is understandable, but so is his or her need to thoroughly understand (McArdle *et al.* 2010). After all, it is important that exercise physiologists thoroughly understand the intricate mix of structure and function of the human body. This thinking requires the study of both anatomy and biochemistry along with numerous other science-oriented courses. One might conclude the same with an increased emphasis on the neurology of weight lifting. However, it should be self-evident that is not the case. Given that the problem seems obvious, it is believed the solution appears to be equally simple.

Yet, the truth is that anatomy has been dropped from the exercise physiology curriculum in favor of other subjects that are more entrenched in physiology (Box **6**). The exercise physiology curriculum is essentially an exercise science and/or sports medicine series of courses that do not address anatomical instruction. Applied anatomy as clinical kinesiology, for example, and gross cadaver-based anatomy are no longer taught. Common sense suggests that this dramatic change of events cannot continue.

Box 6. Exercise physiologist need leadership.

Exercise physiologists need academic leaders who are willing to challenge the status quo. As Gale Baker Stanton said, "To achieve all that is possible, we must attempt the impossible … to be as much as we can be, we must dream of being more."

Since the teaching of exercise physiology applies science to healthcare, the academic major in exercise physiology should emphasize the importance of all the subject areas if students are to understand the human body. This thinking also applies to psychology, self-management and cognitive skills, and the power of one's thinking along with business skills, and beliefs in maintaining and/or developing the integrity of the mind-body complex.

In particular, the failure to delve into the psychophysiology of the client's lifestyle, chronic diseases, and/or disabilities is unacceptable. Students must be prepared to come up with answers for such issues and concerns that arise in regards to the mind-body interconnectedness. Self-management procedures is but one of the many options that need accurate assessment and application to help increase the client's level of function and well-being.

Final Thoughts

Once considered the cornerstone of exercise physiology, applied anatomy is no longer a regular feature in the academic curriculum. This is a problem since non-doctorate exercise physiologists are healthcare professionals first and researchers second. Thus, it is important that they get a thorough academic course in anatomy with application to athletics and healthcare. Failure to teach anatomy impairs the students' ability to: (a) correct and/or enhance the style and execution of regular exercise programs and weight lifting to improve health and wellness; (b) identify appropriate (*i.e.,* good *vs.* useless or dangerous) flexibility exercises to improve range of motion and/or prevent musculoskeletal injuries; and (c) evaluate athletic performance and training programs that require the efficient utilization of the musculoskeletal system.

The anatomy challenge is to put the teaching of anatomy back into the curriculum, and to design teaching strategies to help students develop anatomy vocabulary for articulating anatomical knowledge (Box 7). This means there should be an increased emphasis on the memorization of anatomical facts and the visualization of the musculoskeletal system to understand anatomy.

Box 7. The illusion of a good education.

To date, anatomy is not being taught by exercise physiologists. It would be an exaggeration to suggest otherwise. In coming to terms with this thinking, a college student was heard to say: "Excuse me" – as the look of amused bewilderment came over his face –"Did I hear you say that anatomy is not being taught in exercise physiology and related degree programs? Yes, that is correct. "Why am I just finding out about this? It is news to me! Let me get this right, you are saying that I am a product of a failed system, right? Is that what you are telling me? Isn't the department responsible for teaching all the relevant academic courses to their students? There must be standards as to what constitutes a credible academic degree and for determining unethical behavior. This is very unsettling."

GLOSSARY

Applied anatomy Practical application of anatomical knowledge to diagnosis and treatment and/or specific enhancement of the muscles, bones, and tendons.

Biochemistry Science deals with the chemical processes that occur within living organisms.

Biomechanics Study of the mechanical laws relating to structure and movement of living organisms

Exercise physiologist A healthcare professional who either has an academic degree in exercise physiology or who is certified by ASEP to practice exercise physiology [*via* the Exercise Physiologist Certified exam (EPC)] and, therefore, is recognized as an ASEP Board Certified Exercise Physiologist, or who has a doctorate degree in exercise physiology from an accredited college or university.

Kinesiology Science of human movement.

Physiology Branch of biology that deals with functions of living organisms and their parts.

Visualization Recall or formation of mental visual image.

REFERENCES

Maugham, WS (1915) *Of human bondage,* [Accessed 8th February 2016]. Available from: maugham.thefreelibrary.com/of-human-bondage/54-1

McArdle, WD, Katch, FI & Katch, VL (2010) *Exercise physiology: nutrition, energy, and human performance* Lippincott Williams & Wilkins, New York, New York.

Persaud, TV (1984) *The early history of human anatomy: from antiquity to the beginning of the modern area.* Thomas Books Springfield, Massachusetts.

CHAPTER 2

Why is Anatomy Important?

Abstract: Knowledge of anatomical structure of the body is basic to understanding musculoskeletal function and how both structure and function are modified by exercise or disease. Ironically, at a time when knowledge of anatomy is increasingly important, exercise physiologists are facing a major crisis in anatomical education. There is a major shortage of academic exercise physiologists willing to teach gross anatomy. Many faculty members are simply not academically prepared to teach anatomy. Yet, the students of exercise physiology need a thorough anatomy education to be credible healthcare professionals. This is true for professionals in physical therapy and athletic training and it is true for exercise physiologists too.

Keywords: Anatomical dissection, Athletic performance, Cognitive function, Functional anatomy, Human anatomy, Memorization, Straight thinking.

INTRODUCTION

Several decades ago, the study of the connection between structure and function was considered important. It was common practice for physical education teachers to impress upon their students the importance of learning anatomy and its connection to human performance. Physical education students did not graduate without passing the "kinesiology" course. Understandably, it was considered a difficult course, given that it covered all the major muscles of the body. Also, not all the students enjoy the required memorization of a muscle's origin, insertion, and function.

The Idea is Simple

The original approach to teaching anatomy was simple. If the students could recognize muscles and grasp the connection of one muscle to another, then likelihood of comprehending specific movements and athletic skills would be

Tommy Boone

increased. Since students are interested in sports and athletic performance, they are also interested in academic subjects that allow for an increased understanding skills and physical performance. This was especially the case with anatomy.

The majority of the students had the desire to understand the anatomy of sports skills, and so they rarely ever tried to get out of the course. Every major muscle in the body was memorized, thus raising the issue today. If it was the right thing to do decades ago (*i.e.*, expect students to memorize the origins, insertions, and functions of the muscles of the limbs, why did the history of doing so get lost across time? Was it due to the notion that memorization is not true learning? Or, was it that publishing research papers would help empower the professors' job? Maybe that is why there so little emphasis on the "specifics" of muscles today? It is strange but true that the majority of the exercise physiology and related degrees do not require the students to try something new (Box **1**), like learning applied anatomy? Perhaps, it is as simple as exercise physiologists are not comfortable with trying something new.

Box 1. Try something new.

Never be afraid to try something new. Remember amateurs built the ark. Professionals built the Titanic. -- Author Unknown

To be rather blunt, why doesn't the academic major (whatever its name is, as an offshoot of the original physical education degree) have an anatomy laboratory with cadavers? After all, it is common sense given the perception of the situation college students find themselves in. There is no stand-in for cadaveric analysis in the learning of practical anatomy. Why aren't students taught the importance of visualization skills in learning anatomy? Why is there so little empirical evidence supporting the memorization and visualization in learning anatomy? Why isn't a thorough understanding of anatomy taught to students so that they can learn how to deal with forces that cause athletic injuries and improve human movement?

The Power of Memorization

Without memorization and visualization, it is extremely hard to learn anatomy.

And yet, another part of this chapter is to grasp why anatomy is the missing course in the study of exercise physiology and related academic majors? Perhaps, a piece of the answer rest with the teachers and their students who think that it is a waste of their time to memorize a list of anatomical facts. Others feel that it is utterly irrelevant and boring. Why memorize something when it is so easily forgotten? Memorization is believed to have little to no benefit in learning.

Many college teachers believe that genuine thinking is described as something other than learning by rote. It is said that memorization is useless and unneeded. Or, perhaps, the reader has heard the more common expression. Memorization deflects from a higher measure of intellectual purpose. Although many teachers give the appearance that such statements are actually true, the single largest misconception is the belief that memorization is not important. It is not true that the time put into memorization is pointless. Also, it is increasingly clear that memorization and understanding are vitally important to the learning process (Box **2**). They are not mutually exclusive.

Box 2. Memorization increases cognitive function.

> The memorization and recitation of the classic utterances of poets and statesmen form part of a tradition of learning that stretches back to classical antiquity, when the Greeks discovered that words and sounds — and the rhythmic patterns by which they were bound together in poetry — awakened the mind and shaped character.
>
> -- Michael Knox Beran

To remember different parts of the body that have specific functions, it is important to have an extremely good memory. Many students and professors memorize a considerable volume of subject matter every day. How can students understand the functions of a muscle without knowing its origin and insertion? Similarly, how can students remember physiological calculations without first visualizing the component parts?

Does anyone believe that a person is not as smart as the next person because he or she memorized the Fick equation (VO_2 = Q x a-vO_2 diff)? To understand oxygen consumption (VO_2), students must grasp the significance of cardiac output (Q) and tissue extraction (a-vO_2 diff). Similarly, it isn't likely that a student can fix a musculoskeletal problem without knowing how the muscles and bones work together. Thus, whether it is a physiology formula or the origin and insertion of the pectoralis major muscle (Box **3**) and its functions, remembering the specifics of each is more than having memorized bits of information.

Hence, just as it is necessary for exercise physiology students to know that VO_2 is the product of cardiac output (Q) and oxygen that diffuses from the blood to the tissues (a-vO_2 diff), they need to know that shoulder flexion is the function of four primary shoulder flexors (*i.e.,* the clavicular fibers of the pectoralis major, the anterior deltoid, the coracobrachialis, and the biceps brachii). When looking at the anatomical dissection of the left anterior-lateral chest and abdominal picture, which one of the shoulder flexors is missing without more dissection (Box **3**)? With just a little anatomical insight, it is clear that the shoulder flexor that arises from the coracoid process (coracobrachialis) is the muscle that cannot be seen.

Box 3. Anatomical dissection of the shoulder, chest, and abdominal muscles.

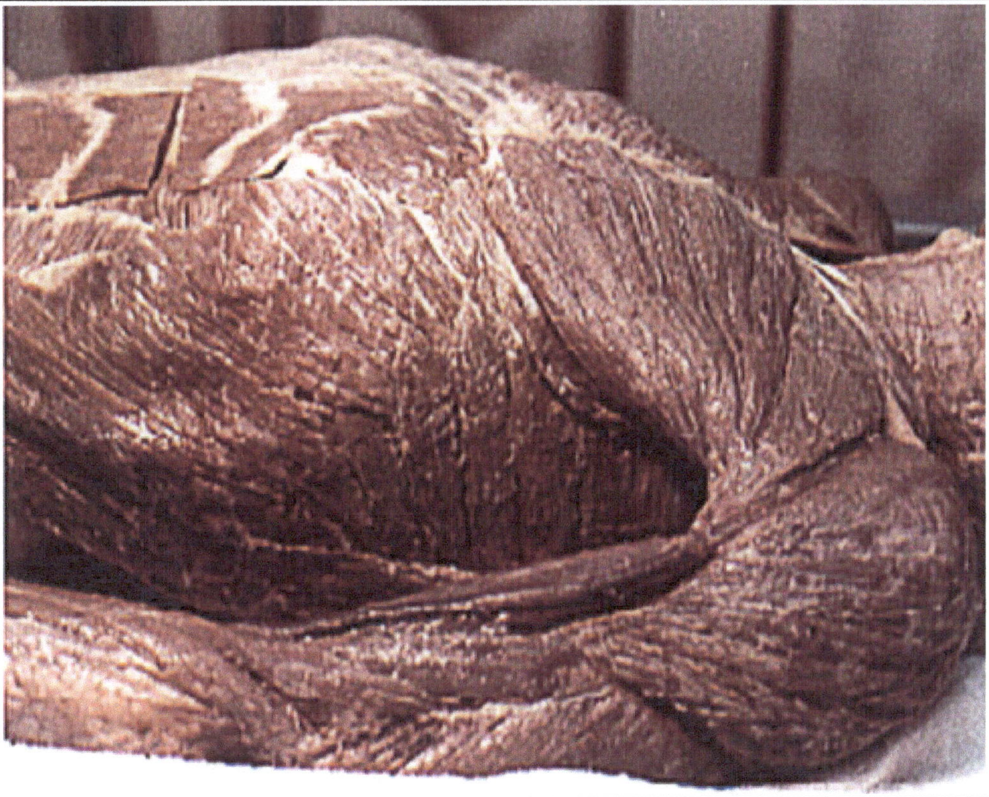

The purpose of memorization is not to recite the points of origin, insertion, and function(s) of a muscle to simply forget the information a short time later. The idea is to acknowledge what is memorized as foundational information that allows for the manipulation of the content to make sense of it in relation to the individual muscle and related muscles and their functions. Without question, rote learning of detailed information is prerequisite to acquiring a deeper meaning and higher quality of learning.

Straight Thinking is Critical

It is not straight thinking to trust that exercise physiologists comprehend the musculoskeletal system without at least a semester-long undergraduate anatomy course (Box **4**). Teachers should know that an appreciation of anatomy is critical to a leadership role in health, fitness, athletic performance, and rehabilitation. If teachers agree this thinking makes sense, it can be argued that anatomy must be taught in the exercise physiology curriculum. They cannot rely on the anatomy and physiology course taught in the biology department. Students do not get the origin, insertion, and function of muscles in the biology course. There is simply too much content that must be introduced, so the description of muscles across the major joints of the body is more of a brief overview.

Box 4. Functional anatomy.

> You can't get as good an education if you don't have access to cadavers for gross anatomy.
>
> -- Len Cleary, PhD
> http://www.uthouston.edu

Also, the notion that anyone can learn anatomy, but only the best, perhaps, the exercise physiologists can learn physiology is not straight thinking. In fact, such reasoning is defective and silly. It sets the stage for disagreement in particular with colleagues in sports training, athletics, and human movement. Such a disturbing perspective is not only troublesome it is atypical of the professional status of the professors.

While there is little written on this point, it appears to have a relationship to the fact that applied anatomy is not part of the exercise physiology curriculum at the doctorate level. There are only a small number of exercise physiology programs that require a gross anatomy course with cadavers. Think of the shortcoming of the PhD degree that is focused on the human body and yet, the future professors finalize their schooling without a functional anatomy course much less the opportunity to work with cadavers. It is the same incorrectness as in trying to study the physiology of VO_2 max without having the opportunity to measure it with a metabolic analyzer, cycle ergometer, and/or treadmill.

Academic exercise physiologists understand the need for the innovative metabolic analyzers and other physiological paraphernalia to identify with physiology. The vision to procure cadavers from appropriate medical facilities from which human donations are received for a more thorough trustworthy instruction and analysis of human anatomy does not appear to pierce their intellect. Unquestionably, the significance of knowing anatomy that is equal to one's knowledge of physiology is not hard to understand.

A 21st century anatomy laboratory for exercise physiology students makes all the sense in the world (Box **5**). It would not be all that difficult to provide hands-on lab instruction with a faculty to student ratio of 1:20 at an average student to cadaver ratio of 5:1 (given an average expense of $1000 per cadaver for a total investment of $5000 per academic year). But, first, what about the availability of instructors from within the exercise physiology faculty? That is the problem! Who is going to oversee the Anatomy Laboratory and cadaver dissection?

Box 5. Accreditation and gross anatomy.

Except for the ASEP accreditation guidelines, there is no national requirement for exercise physiology related academic programs to teach anatomy. Hence, they are free to teach or not to teach anatomy. When it comes to actual learning, digital is not equal to cadavers.

Recapturing the Original Thinking

Why teach the science of anatomy to exercise physiology students? It is enough to know how to develop muscle strength, right? How about the development of the muscular endurance? The two topics are connected, aren't they? Or, is it as simple as anatomy is irrelevant (*i.e.,* nothing left to discover)? Really, what about the recent report of the anterolateral ligament of the knee (Claes *et al.* 2013)?

An understanding of anatomical structures, connective tissues, articulations, muscles, and nerves should be part of the exercise physiologist's assessment of a client. Despite the unanswered anatomical questions mentioned earlier, it is necessary that Board Certified Exercise Physiologists recapture the original view of human movement as a synthesis of many interactions. This point is highlighted by the integrated involvement of the musculoskeletal system, nervous system, kinematics of human function, and organic chemistry of movement in general.

Cadavers are used in healthcare professions either for hands-on anatomical dissection, prosection, or a combination of both. It makes sense that this should be done in exercise physiology. The opportunity to study dissected cadavers deepens the students' understanding of anatomic structures. Dissected cadaver-based anatomy is better than computers, plastic models, and other teaching tools. The teaching of anatomy must be improved (Older 2004). It serves to help link the healthcare opportunities for exercise physiologists with other professionals in the public sector. Thus, a sound knowledge of dissected anatomy (Box **6**) is essential if exercise physiologists are going to accurately define and treat health problems presented by their clients.

Box 6. Abdominal dissection.

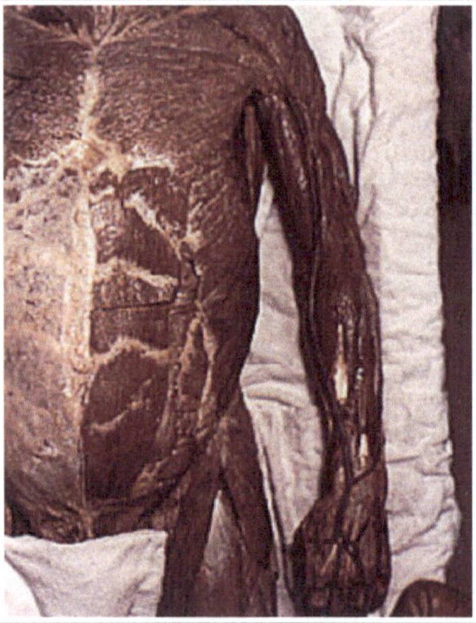

The failure to teach anatomy has led to college students graduating without a meaningful understanding of the human body. For example, with the opportunity to dissect the abdominal wall, students have a much greater appreciation for the correct exercises. After removal of the rectus sheath on the left side, note the four tendinous intersections that divide the muscle that runs vertical on each side of the anterior abdominal wall (*i.e.,* the rectus abdominis). In this case, they divide the muscle into five functional parts. Note the external oblique that passes anterior to the rectus abdominis to end at the linea alba. The insertion of the internal oblique takes place by passing anterior and posterior to the rectus abdominis to also insert at the linea alba. The transversus abdominis is the deep fourth abdominal muscle. It, too, inserts into the linea alba.

An appreciation of functional anatomy is also necessary to acquiring knowledge of the human body in sports and fitness. For example, what are the white lines that run across the rectus abdominis? Why are the lines important? How do the oblique muscles relate anatomically to the abdominal wall? Is it true that lying on the back and lifting the legs is the best way to develop the abdominal muscles? If so, what is the role of the psoas major and iliacus muscles in hip flexion?

Ironically, the obvious lack of emphasis in teaching anatomy can be reverse. But, first exercise physiologists must place a greater emphasis on anatomical skills and human development. This can be accomplished by expanding the meaning of research to include an increased commitment to the teaching of gross anatomy, particularly at the doctorate level. As a result, there would be more doctorate prepared exercise physiologists with training in cadaver anatomy and experience in dissection to teach anatomy. Cadavers should be obtained from a medical school and placed the Anatomy Laboratory of the Department of Exercise Physiology. Department chairs should encourage the academic integration of the physiological lectures with the teaching of gross anatomy.

Functional Anatomy

The solution to understanding anatomy comes from anatomy itself. For example, take the picture of the posterior leg (Box **7**). Is it the soleus or the gastrocnemius that is primarily responsible for plantar flexor? In short, what is it about the soleus muscle that makes it the "powerhouse" of the plantar flexors? Why isn't the two-headed muscle that arises above the knee joint to insert on the dorsal surface of the calcaneus the primary plantar flexor? Knowledge of anatomy helps the students understand the specifics of different weight training practices.

If exercise physiologists are to assist with the professionalization of exercise physiologists, it is imperative that they promote the teaching of anatomy at all academic levels of the students' education. The functional anatomy course is more important to the students of exercise physiology than another course in physiology, biomechanics, or nutrition. There is something unsound with the idea of exercise physiologists doing muscle fiber research who cannot pinpoint the four nerves to the shoulder flexors and abductors. This is but one reason why the problem must be corrected. We owe it to the future to help ensure that exercise physiologists are taught by college teachers with an in-depth knowledge of and appreciation for functional anatomy.

Box 7. The posterior view of the right leg.

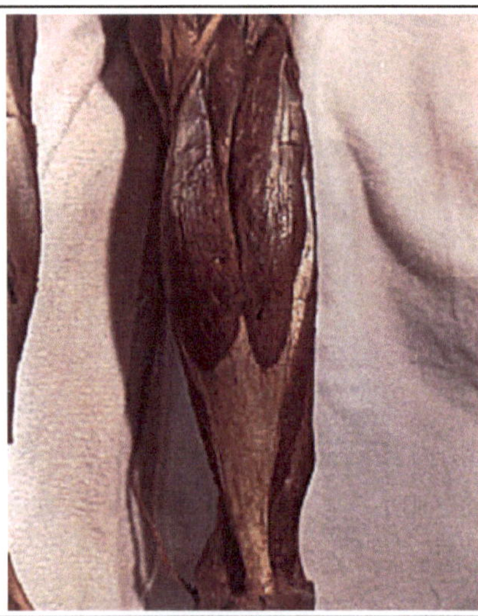

The **gastrocnemius** is the most superficial muscle in the posterior part of the leg. It arises from the medial and lateral condyles of the femur and inserts on the posterior surface of the calcaneus. It flexes the leg at the knee joint and plantar flexes the foot.

The **soleus** is located deep to the gastrocnemius. It is a large one-joint muscle arising from the proximal posterior aspects of the fibula and tibia to insert on the calcaneus with the gastrocnemius. The soleus is the workhorse of the plantar flexors. You can see the soleus on medial and lateral sides of the calcaneal tendon.

Anatomy was for decades one of the important cornerstones of understanding and teaching health and fitness. The study of anatomy of the living body is certainly as important as students learning the cellular enzymes for energy production. Ultimately, the knowledge that comes from the study of anatomy (such as the medial pectoral nerve innervates the sternal fibers of the pectoralis major and the pectoralis minor, as in shoulder extension and downward rotation of the scapula, respectively) allows for the understanding of human movement that is equally important as in knowing the histologic differences between fiber types.

This thinking is supported by both the necessity to memorize and visualize the intricate parts of the human body. The point is this: The memorized information must be used. The objective is not the memorization, but the visual transition to understanding the positive anatomical relationship of the pectoralis minor muscle to the rhomboid major and rhomboid minor. In short, this thinking is the same as holding a baseball in one's hand and knowing how to throw it. Clearly, if the ball is never thrown, there is little incentive for understanding the purpose behind the ball (*i.e.,* that of playing a baseball game).

Anatomical Knowledge

Applied anatomy should be the signature course of the undergraduate exercise physiology curriculum. Structure sets the stage for function. Exercise physiology is all about function, especially the contributions to the physiology of athletics and sports training (Box **8**). Exercise physiology should also be about making sense of and remembering well-designed visual images of the body in motion. That is why a required course in anatomy and its connection to the profession of exercise physiology are important. Thus, for that reason, exercise physiologists should teach osteology to their students so they can understand the points of origin and insertion of the muscles, the myology required to grasp the relationship of muscles of different joints, and the neurology that is necessary to appreciate the role of the nervous system in human movement. In addition, it is imperative that specific joint motions are analyzed with reference to joint-specific muscles and their relationship and functions across one-joint or two-joints and how each singly or collectively produces the desired musculoskeletal movement.

Box 8. The ASEP definition of exercise physiology.

"The comprehensive delivery of treatment services concerned with the analysis, improvement, and maintenance of the physiological mechanisms underlying physical and mental health and fitness through regular exercise, the rehabilitation of heart disease and other chronic diseases and/or disabilities with exercise medicine, and the professional guidance of athletes and others interested in athletics and sports training" (American Society of Exercise Physiologists 2016).

The anatomical analysis can take on numerous forms, such as weight training, sports skills analysis, fitness development, and rehabilitation. The joints and the range of motion possible should be understood in terms of the nervous system and, in particular, the specific link between the central nervous system and the peripheral nervous system. Students should be taught the anatomical specifics of the brachial plexus and upper extremity motion. They need to understand the role of the lumbosacral plexus in lower extremity motion. Students should be taught the spinal nerves that innervate skeletal muscles so that they can fully understand the loss in muscle function. The nerve and muscle connection is vital to a firm scientific knowledge in any science-oriented academic degree that gives rise to the students' responsibility for improving the human body, either in the athletic world of preparing athletes to perform or as a function of managing the client's muscular system to improve lifestyle for a better quality of life.

Exercise physiologists trained in anatomy are prepared to produce, modify, and/or restore the prerequisites and appropriate hands-on rehabilitative skills necessary to help athletic achieve success. The method and technique of athletic function cannot be ascertained, coached, or developed without the insight derived from an appreciation of the complex language of the structure of the body. Without question, anatomy is equal in significance to the study of physiology, and it is indivisible from exercise physiology in that anatomy helps to define physiology.

The Physical Education Connection

Although exercise physiology is for the most part separated from its historical connections to physical education, one of the trademarks of the physical education degree has always been the "kinesiology" course that provided anatomy to the students. Every health and physical education student was required to pass a semester of applied anatomy (*i.e.,* kinesiology). As a result, it was believed that the students would graduate with an in-depth understanding of the anatomical knowledge to safely promote health and fitness programs. The idea itself goes back for many decades (Houglum & Bertoti 2012; Jensen & Schultz 1970; Rasch & Burke 1971).

Over time, to promote the science way of thinking more so than the activity approach to the physical education degree, the physical education degree title was changed across many academic departments to "kinesiology" (*i.e.,* the science of movement). Physical educators became known as kinesiologists or "exercise scientists" (Box **9**). Interestingly, regardless of the title, the academic course, kinesiology, gradually disappeared from the curriculum. Departments became known by dozens of different titles with students graduating without a meaningful career-driven opportunity in the public sector (Rademacher & Pittsley, 2001).

Today, many of these academic programs have minimal emphasis on applied anatomy. While there are several considerations, the primary reason exists with the increased concerns for sports biomechanics decades ago (Duvall 1959). In short, physical educators were perplexed, that is not knowing for sure which to teach – they chose biomechanics over anatomy to analyze human movement (Dyson 1962; Hall 1995; Hay 1985). Their influence has had a negative effect on the anatomical knowledge of students due to the lack of emphasis in teaching the kinesiology course. Professors with an interest in biomechanics introduced new technological equipment that allowed for instant data collection.

Box 9. Exercise science *vs.* sports science and human performance.

One student asked another, what is your major? He said, Exercise Science. And you, John: Your major is what? Did you say, Sports Sciences? Yes, but I'm thinking of finding another university to major in Health and Human Performance. Are you sure? What is that? I think it is the same as Exercise Science. All of these different majors sound like the system is messed up to me. What do you think? Frankly, I haven't thought about it.

In short, the interest in anatomy has been replaced by the idea that biomechanics is the upcoming science. While the introduction of biomechanics is important, this reasoning presented a change in the physical educator's thinking about good and/or bad movement. It is difficult to comprehend why the striking turn of events was permitted to occur much less continue unabated. As a result, the typical academic kinesiology course today is often a combination of both basic anatomy and applied biomechanics. In some of these academic programs, the teaching of biomechanics has completed replaced kinesiology and any thoughts regarding anatomy.

Why? There are primarily two reasons:

1. With the advances in technological equipment, the physical education and exercise science faculty had increased access to biomechanical data that set the stage for publishing more research papers.
2. Anatomy requires students to memorize content, which was then (and still is today) believed by many academics to be a poor way to learn subject content.

While there are strong reasons to teach students biomechanical principles, none of them is adequate in the displacement of teaching anatomical knowledge. Students who intend to prescribe exercise medicine to prevent and treat chronic diseases and disabilities need to have a thorough understanding of the human body and its functions. That is why the capacity to think 3-dimensionally about muscle structure and function are so important. It provides the opportunity to see the anatomy of the human body in "real time" either at rest or in motion that leads to important and relevant decisions suitable to all exercise physiology careers.

Final Thoughts

Anatomy has been a cornerstone of students with an interest in health, fitness, and athletics. However, in recent decades, human anatomy has been displaced by the increased emphasis placed on biomechanics and physiology-oriented courses. Why are the academic exercise physiologists participating in this change in the curriculum? The primary reason appears to be the lack of emphasis on anatomy in their doctoral programs. Also, many faculty members argue that publishing research papers is a more effective way to advance in academia than spending hours after hours teaching dissection to their students in an anatomy laboratory. Of course, the reality is that only a few exercise physiology departments actually have their own cadaver laboratory.

As an educator and healthcare professional, it is increasingly clear that there are litigious factors supporting the need to teach exercise physiology students the anatomical and physiological knowledge they need to safely prescribe exercise medicine. This is true regardless of the cost factor in terms of paying for the cadavers and staff as well as the relatively small faculty to student ratio per cadaver? In fact, there is no reason that the cost of cadavers and maintaining a dissection laboratory should be viewed differently from the typical expenses associated with purchasing and maintaining metabolic carts, treadmills, cycle ergometers, and/or other standard pieces of laboratory equipment. Obviously, what is important is what is best for the students.

As with any curriculum change, it must be inventive, progressive, and credible. Students' education in exercise physiology must be the best it can be. This means that the academic infrastructure, curriculum, and emphasis on anatomy should be updated. Therefore, the question that must be answered is this: "Will the exercise physiology faculty provide the best educational experience for their students?" As a spin-off from this question, there is also the concern of the department chair and other administrators and their support of the exercise physiology educators.

Given all this, isn't there a moral context to teaching as well? That is, is it not logical to conclude that teaching should always be about the students and their well-being? If so, why are the academic exercise physiologists continuing to keep things as they have been when change is imperative? Surely, they must know that a degree without a connection to professionalism is not a credible attempt in helping students find a job after college (Box **10**).

Box 10. Are you a professional?

Think about it. Are you a professional? This might seem like an unnecessary question at first, but have you taken the time to think about it? This is exactly what the members of the American Society of Exercise Physiologists have done. It is more than simply getting an academic degree. The road to professionalism starts with the professional organization. It is everything, especially given its responsibility for academic credibility, accountability, altruism, integrity, compassion, professional duty, excellence, and social responsibility.

GLOSSORY

Anatomical dissection	Process of cutting or separating tissue to study *anatomy.*
Athletic performance	Execution of a routine (such as gymnastics) or procedures required of a particular sport or physical activity.
Cognitive function	A mental process by which a person becomes aware of new ideas, perception, and/or comprehension of information and knowledge.
Functional anatomy	Study of anatomy in its relationship to the specifics of different muscles, skeletal parts, and/or organ function.
Human anatomy	Study of the structure of the human body.
Litigious	Tending, ready, or eager to sue (*i.e.*, take legal action to settle disputes) in a court of law.
Memorization	To commit to memory.
Straight thinking	Thinking that is clear and using good judgment.

REFERENCES

American Society of Exercise Physiologists. What is exercise physiology, [Online], https://www.asep.org/index.php/about-asep/definition/.

Claes, S, Vereecke, E, Maes, M, Victor, J, Verdonk, P & Bellemans, J (2013) Anatomy of the anterolateral ligament of the knee *Journal of Anatomy,* 223, 321-8. [Online], http://www.ncbi.nlm.nih.gov/pubmed/23906341.

Duvall, EN (1959) *Kinesiology: the anatomy of motion.* Prentice-Hall, Inc, Englewood Cliffs, New Jersey.

Dyson, GH (1962) *The mechanics of athletics.* University of London Press Ltd, England.

Hall, SJ (1995) *Basic biomechanics.* McGraw-Hill, Boston, Massachusetts.

Hay, JG (1985) *The biomechanics of sports techniques.* Prentice-Hall, Inc, Englewood Cliffs, New Jersey.

Houglum, PA & Bertoti, DB (2012) *Brunnstrom's clinical kinesiology* F. A. Davis Company, Philadelphia, Pennsylvania.

Jensen, C & Schultz, GW (1970) *Applied kinesiology: the scientific study of human performance.* McGraw-Hill Book Company, New York, NY.

Older, J (2004) Anatomy: a must for teaching the next generation. *Surgeon,* 2, 79-90. [http://dx.doi.org/10.1016/S1479-666X(04)80050-7] [PMID: 15568432]

Rademacher, E & Pittsley, J (2001) Analysis and comparison of colleges and universities with degree titles of exercise physiology or related titles *Professionalization of Exercise Physiologyonline,* 4 [Online], http://www.css.edu/users/tboone2/asep/MinimalStandards.html

Rasch, PJ & Burke, RK (1971) *Kinesiology and applied anatomy: the science of human movement.* Lea and Febiger, Philadelphia, Pennsylvania.

CHAPTER 3

Shortage of Qualified Instructors

Abstract: Given the presence of so many educated men and women today, one would expect that there would be a sufficient number of anatomy teachers. Point in fact though, there are too few healthcare professionals with a credible knowledge of and actual hands-on laboratory experiences in anatomy instruction and application to human movement and healthcare. While there are numerous reasons why anatomy is no longer taught in exercise physiology and related degree programs, one in particular is the cost, time, and challenges to maintain a dissection room. Another reason is the unsupportive academic infrastructure. None of these reasons is justified. Anatomy is obviously essential for exercise physiologists as credible healthcare professionals.

Keywords: Core curriculum, Healthcare professional, Integrity, Muscle function, Muscle insertion, Muscle origin.

INTRODUCTION

Knowledge of the structure of the human body is imperative for career success. There is no substitute for not achieving mastery of the subject. While the non-doctorate exercise physiologists do not need to know anatomy at the molecular level, they do need to know functional anatomy. Otherwise, how will they know what is safe and appropriate in developing individualized weight lifting and/or flexibility exercises to maintain health and fitness?

To understand the present situation, it is necessary to highlight the fact that doctorate prepared exercise physiologists do not take a gross anatomy course and know nothing about dissection. Also, they are not taught the methods of 3-D awareness that helps them conceptualize and visualize anatomy. Worse yet, they have little to no knowledge as to how they should teach anatomy or connect basic and clinical issues that pertain to regular exercise training, health, and wellness to

Tommy Boone

their exercise physiology students. For further progress to be made professionally speaking, the administration and faculty members must concede that anatomy is necessary in the exercise physiology curriculum.

A Credible Education is Important

Imagine this: A recent college graduate was hired to supervise the development of a muscular strength training program for high school athletes. On the first day, he entered into a conversation with the head football coach regarding the specifics of different weight lifting exercises to help decrease the frequency of injuries to specific muscles and joints and to significantly strengthen certain other muscles. To the coach's surprise, the discussion did not go well. When he asked about specific exercises to build certain muscles, the coach realized that the new hire did not have knowledge of anatomy or an understanding of which exercises would be better than others. Then, the coach said, "You did take an anatomy class in college, right?" The new hire said, "No, none of my teachers knew how to teach anatomy (Box **1**)".

Box 1. Difficulty in finding anatomy teachers.

> In a survey conducted by the American Association of Anatomists, it was noted that 83% of heads of departments had great or moderate difficulty in the recruitment of qualified gross anatomy teachers.
>
> -- American Association of Anatomists (2002)

Without an understanding of the human body, its actual parts, and how they relate to each other, it is essentially impossible to rely on an exercise physiologist (or anyone for that matter) to produce the right results. Every exercise physiologist must understand the origin, insertion, and function of muscles just as they are expected to know the rate-limiting enzymes of glycolysis or that cardiac output is the volume of blood the left ventricle pumps every minute. Ironically, at a time when knowledge of anatomy is important, students are graduating with a huge void in their education. It does not help that exercise physiologists understand the role hemoglobin plays in providing oxygen to the muscles if they do not understand the functional differences in the brachialis and the biceps brachii.

The lack of experienced exercise physiologists to teach anatomical knowledge threatens the integrity of the profession. It is for this reason alone that changes in the education of exercise physiologists in the United States must improve. This is true at all levels of education, from the undergraduate degree through the doctorate program. Here, the point is that it is not a question of developing new methods to examine the molecular or genetic basis of cellular function. What is important is the knowledge of the human body. For example, how muscles work, how they move, and what is normal function? Having such knowledge will help the Board Certified Exercise Physiologist to better understand the application of exercise medicine.

Will cadavers cost the department? Yes, that is correct. Just as there is an expense to purchase metabolic carts and all the other rather common pieces of equipment in an exercise physiology laboratory, there is a cost factor. But, the expenses are necessary to expanding the department's professional infrastructure and the quality of the students' education. It is especially important that academic exercise physiologists understand this point, just as they realize that the physiology equipment is required to teach the students about the physiological functions of the body with increased clarity and precision. Hence, while faculty-centered didactic lectures are important, students are in a much better position to compete with other healthcare students when they have access to a qualified teacher with a cadaver-based anatomical education and experience (Box **2**).

Box 2. Qualified anatomy instructors.

Many exercise physiologists don't want to teach anatomy because it demands roughly twice as much time as other academic courses and yet, it is essential to the exercise physiology students' education. The bottom line is this: No exposure to dissection and dissected specimens is likely to compromise future exercise physiologists, which is also a recipe for malpractice.

Benefits of Teaching Anatomy

Learning by direct observation sets the path for creative and critical thinking. Just as Leonardo da Vinci and Michelangelo studied anatomy from cadavers to help them create impressive works of art, exercise physiology professors should study anatomy from cadavers to become the best professionals they can be. Those who will benefit from the teaching of anatomy will be their students, clients, and patients.

As academic departments advertise the anatomy course to reflect the expanded thinking and teaching activities of the faculty and students, there will be an increase in the flow of students to those departments with the effect of helping to reduce the existence of programs where anatomy isn't taught. As the students graduate and search for careers in healthcare to experience an even greater sense of "what is" applied anatomy, they will eventually become the new faculty members who will be hired for their anatomical knowledge and expertise. It is they who will show the exercise physiologist's unique application of exercise and human anatomy to health, wellness, rehabilitation, and sports training.

In time with the adoption of an exercise physiology core curriculum that defines fundamental knowledge necessary for a credible exercise physiology practice, students will be prepared to apply anatomical concepts equally as well as they do physiology concepts. However, this raises two important points. Firstly, there must be a common rationale for students to have knowledge of anatomy in exercise physiology. Secondly, the academic exercise physiologists must then emphasize the teaching and anatomical dissection of anatomy (Box **3**).

Box 3. Anatomy training is essential.

Anatomy education is not only an essential part of the profession of exercise physiology, it is critical to the educational development and professionalism of Board Certified Exercise Physiologists. This point is so important that the American Society of Exercise Physiologists made sure that an "anatomy" course was listed among the exercise physiology courses required to graduate from an ASEP accredited academic institution. For example, students must be able to (American Society of Exercise Physiologists 2016):

- Demonstrate proper anatomical terminology associated with body structures, directional location, and movement;
- Identify skeletal and joint structures and demonstrate knowledge of their function in human movement;
- Identify and explain the movement function of muscles including their origin, insertion, and action singly and collectively;
- Demonstrate knowledge of other anatomical structures that are vital to human movement (such as the brachial plexus and lumbosacral plexus); and
- Identify joint movements and which muscles are involved and what their specific roles are in complex human movements.

Remember that such thinking is the outcome of what was once understood as "required teaching" and, therefore, was not questioned decades ago. To a substantial degree, the result of this reform will be a dramatic increase in time and content of gross anatomical instruction and knowledge. Obviously, this means that the instructional time for anatomy will increase as will the number of exercise physiologists trained to teach anatomy.

Since the majority of the doctorate prepared exercise physiologists work in academia and do research, more often than not they need extramural funding for research equipment and other laboratory considerations. Having a good record of publishing also helps in securing grant funds and getting promoted and/or tenured. The changes in health and physical education to kinesiology, exercise science, human performance, and exercise physiology have not altered the academic environment, its focus, and the emphasis placed on doing research. What has changed is the diminished emphasis on teaching anatomy and its application to athletics and healthcare in exercise physiology.

Both anatomists and healthcare professionals agree that an accurate knowledge of anatomy is vital to the students' practice after graduation. Also, from a clinical perspective, it helps to decrease the likelihood of errors irrespective of the healthcare profession. Hence, regardless of the time and/or money constraints, it is imperative that college administrators correct the shortage of faculty qualified to teach anatomy.

The Shortage Problem

But, unless the exercise physiology faculty talk about anatomy with the same passion as they typically do for other exercise physiology courses (*e.g.,* sports nutrition, biomechanics, exercise prescription, ECG/graded exercise testing), students are not likely to experience the benefits of knowing anatomy. They will not get the message that it is fundamental to understanding bodily function and how both structure (anatomy) and function (physiology) are modified by the specifics of origin and insertion of muscles singly and collectively (Box **4**).

When they are hired as an exercise physiologist, and the Department Chair says, "You are going to teach an anatomy course this spring." The new hire is likely to say, "No, I cannot do that. Actually, no, I really cannot teach the class. I was not taught anatomy in doctorate school. Moreover, it would take time away from my research, which is what I do."

Box 4. Anatomical dissection of the posterior leg.

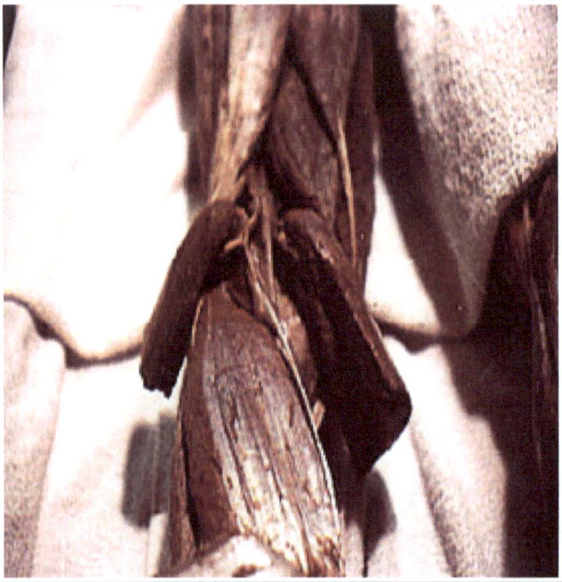

Note that the **gastrocnemius** muscle has been cut across its middle, which allows for seeing the **soleus** muscle under it. As a one-joint muscle, the soleus is a powerful plantar flexor of the ankle. Also, note that the **plantaris** muscle with its short belly and a long tendon can be seen on top and to the medial side of the soleus muscle. The plantaris is absent in 5 to 10% of people, and it is highly variable in size and form when present. It acts with the gastrocnemius but is essentially insignificant as a flexor of the knee and/or a plantar flexor of the ankle. The merging (and the insertion) of the gastrocnemius and soleus muscles are often called the triceps surae muscle, given the insertion of the three-headed muscle on the calcaneus.

Even if the new hire is bold enough to get prepared to teach anatomy, eventually there will be the realization that teaching an anatomy course will be time intensive. Aside from the time it takes to understand individual muscles, there will be additional time spent learning how to speak and apply anatomy to athletics and healthcare. If there is an anatomy laboratory component, it will usually last approximately five hours in duration once a week. This far exceeds the time other faculty members will spend in the typical exercise physiology laboratory.

The shortage of exercise physiologists who can teach anatomy has come at a time when knowledge of anatomy is increasingly important. Yet, finding qualified faculty to teach anatomy is next to impossible. That is why college teachers with a sports biomechanics background are asked to teach anatomy. Unfortunately, their knowledge of the structure of the human body is poor as well.

Neither the typical biomechanist nor the exercise physiologist would be prepared to correctly identify the two tendons posterior to the lateral malleolus (Box **5**) much less the four tendons on the dorsal side of the distal leg and foot (from medial to lateral) and which two of the four tendons do not insert on the distal phalanges of the five toes.

Box 5. Anatomical dissection of the lateral aspect of the ankle and dorsal foot.

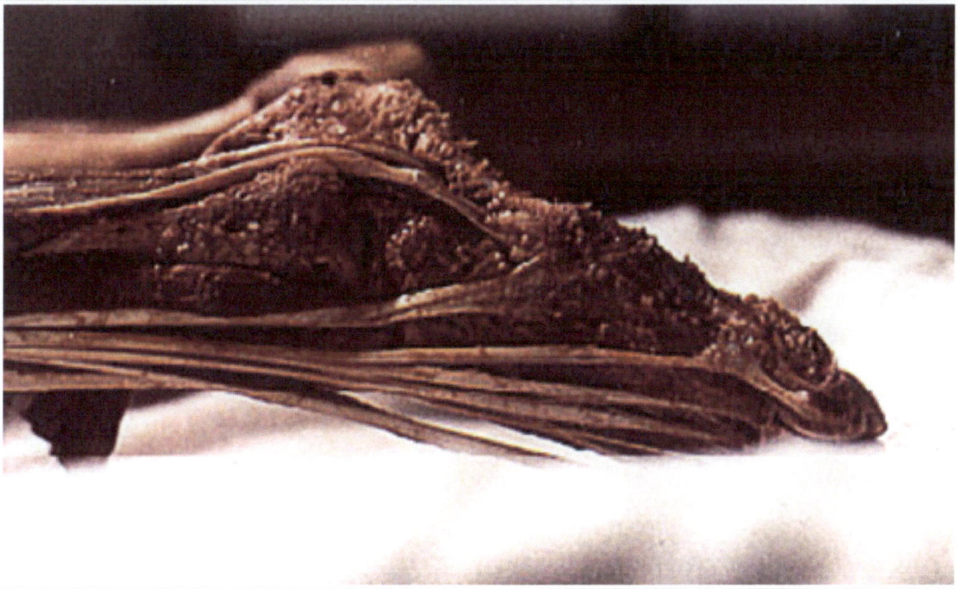

If exercise physiologists choose not to address this problem, they risk producing a generation of healthcare professionals whose knowledge of human structure and function comes primarily from instructors who learned human anatomy "just in time to teach today's lecture". Interestingly, this is very likely why there is an interest in the CD technology used in some classes to teach anatomy.

Final Thoughts

The academic exercise physiologist is not prepared to teach anatomy. Indeed, during the last 30 years, the majority of the universities in the United States have abandoned anatomy as a major subject in exercise physiology. It is apparent that the exercise physiology professors have little knowledge and hands-on experience necessary to teach gross anatomy to exercise physiology students.

This shortage of faculty qualified to teach anatomy is problematic. Students need the exposure to well-trained faculty members. The professional challenge is to update the doctorate programs in exercise physiology so that they offer anatomy to graduates who can become the teachers needed to educate the next generation of exercise physiologists as healthcare professionals (Box **6**).

This is an academic problem, especially since new faculty members are often hired for their research strengths and not for their training or interest in teaching anatomy and/or directing an anatomy laboratory. Also, the obvious fact of not having the requisite knowledge of anatomy and the hands-on dissection skills to teach anatomy distract from exercise physiologists as healthcare professionals.

Box 6. Shortage of qualified teachers of anatomy.

> There can be no questioning of the fact that one of the outstanding problems of the future will be that of finding sufficient suitable staff for the teaching of anatomy.
>
> -- Denis Dooley
> Arris and Gale Lecture delivered on May 10, 1972.

GLOSSORY

Core curriculum	Set of academic courses that are considered essential for education, graduation, employment, and credibility.
Healthcare professional	Person who provides preventive or rehabilitative healthcare services in a systematic way to individuals.
Integrity	Adherence to moral and ethical principles.
Muscle function	Generate force to perform specific actions or functions.
Muscle insertion	The muscle's insertion moves with contraction.
Muscle origin	The muscle's origin is generally a fixed attachment to bone.

REFERENCES

American Association of Anatomists, Association of Anatomy, Cell Biology, and Neurobiology Chairpersons. Survey of academic departments related to anatomy, [Online], http://www.anatomy.org/Membership/survey_academic_departments.htm

American Society of Exercise Physiologists Accreditation of Exercise Physiology. [Online], https://www.asep.org/index.php/professional-services/accreditation/

Dooley, D (1972) A dissection of anatomy: from the Arris and Gale Lecture delivered on 10th May 1972

Annals of The Royal College of Surgeons of England, 53, 13-26. [Online], http://www.ncbi.nlm.nih.gov/pmc/articles/PMC2388318/pdf/annrcse00843-0019.pdf

CHAPTER 4

Teaching Anatomy

Abstract: Anatomy is the study of the structures of the body. Physiology is the study of the function of the structures. The study of both provides a solid understanding of the body and how to develop it and rehabilitate it. There is a great divergence in exercise physiology departments in teaching exercise physiology in general and anatomy in particular. Exercise physiologists must not be disempowered from anatomy. To not have the power to influence the profession would be an appalling state of affairs. Yet, it is clear that students are graduating without knowing in detail which muscles are responsible for what actions.

Keywords: Academic preparation, Hands-on dissection, Language of anatomy, Meaningless stretching exercises, Science of physiology.

INTRODUCTION

When anatomy is not taught, there is little opportunity to understand anatomical principles and relationships. The decrease in anatomical content has led to an insufficient anatomical foundation that creates anxiety because of the perception of not being prepared. If the client's safety comes first, it is imperative that exercise physiologists know anatomy. This thinking should not come as a surprise because anatomy has always been an essential knowledge for healthcare professionals. Thus, it should be inseparable from physiology in that anatomical structure reflects physiology.

Have you examined the students' concerns when they have little to no access to anatomy in their curriculum? They are not comfortable with the notion of mortgaging their future to the whim of a law suit. The volume of anatomical knowledge that students should know but are not being taught is significant. Part of the problem stems from the idea that exercise physiology is said to be all about

Tommy Boone

physiology. After all, physiology is part of the "exercise physiology" title. But, there are no academic programs or professional titles for "exercise anatomy" or for the "exercise anatomy professional". Perhaps, there should be (Box **1**).

Box 1. The visionary!

"…the prophet is the visionary who imagines a desirable future and then declares it to the rest of the world." -- Terry Pearce *Leading Out Loud*

The vision and rationale for studying anatomy at the same level as studying physiology exist only in the judgment of a few exercise physiologists. Even more disconcerting, when anatomy is taught, it is clear that the majority of the exercise physiology faculty either lacks the academic preparation to teach anatomy or has no interest in doing so. Frankly, there is little incentive to teach gross anatomy.

Interestingly, Paalman (2000) points out "that the structure of the human form is being emphasized less and less…." It tends to be scant at worse and patchy at best. The fundamentals of applied anatomy are not being taught in the exercise physiology curriculum? If students express an interest in anatomy, teachers may refer them to the internet or an interactive anatomy software package, which only promotes the crisis we now face.

This brings up an interesting and overarching point of some faculty members. That is, the domain of what is often termed general anatomy in contrast to specific anatomy. In short, it has been said, "Why not stop with the memorization of origin and insertion? Exercise physiologists are not medical doctors! All they need is the practical knowledge of surface anatomy." This thinking is not new and, frankly, it is completely a wrong way to think.

Such thinking seems to be related to medicine's reliance on magnetic resonance imaging (MRI), computerized tomography (CT scan), and positron emission tomography (PET). The problem with such thinking is that many patients expect their primary care doctors to have a detailed command of anatomical structure and the technological means to obtain a detailed understanding of an intact body. The same thinking is (or should be) true for the exercise physiology professional.

The public sector would be startled to know how little knowledge of anatomical structures many healthcare practitioners have. They would be even more shocked to learn that the interactive DVD-Drive has replaced the anatomy laboratory. In fact, the evidence supports the trend of decreased time on cadaver dissection and of increased time on technology-based instruction. The impression is that today's physicians view their education resulting from the hot ticket items, which are very frequently expensive ways to identify an illness or dysfunction. Increasingly sophisticated equipment and technology are used to teach the essentials of anatomy, which is a problem for many doctoral students.

The new modalities (*e.g.,* plastic models, computers, and other diagnostic tools), imaging technologies (including the interactive functional anatomy DVDs), and body painting are giving shape to a new kind of an anatomy experience. Unless these cadaver free approaches are challenged or properly integrated with traditional cadaveric dissection, the future of anatomy will exist entirely in the classroom. The familiarity with real-time hands-on dissection experiences (Box **2**) will be pushed to side for computer course-specific-assisted instruction (CAI) modules (Reidenberg & Laitman 2002).

Box 2. 3-dimensional anatomy *vs.* hands-on cadaver anatomy.

"You can only do so much with a computer. To train properly, there is no substitute for a cadaver," said Eric Reichman, PhD, MD, director of the Surgical and Clinical Skills Center and associate professor of emergency medicine. "Some medical schools are supplementing cadavers with computers and reducing the number of cadavers, but it's not good — especially for spatial training. You can look at a cadaver and see where a muscle starts and ends and what's around it. You need to be able to see it 3-D and feel it."

--http://www.uthouston.edu/Media/newsreleases/nr2007/grossanatomy.htm

The challenge for educators is to not walk away from anatomy, but rather to expand the curriculum accordingly to teach human anatomy to the students of exercise physiology at all levels. There should be no debate or disagreement on this point, given that anatomy still has a place in educating students. A sound knowledge of anatomy is essential if the profession of exercise physiology is going to accurately define and successfully work with clients.

Exercise Physiologists need Anatomy

There isn't any question exercise physiologists need to study bodily structure. An exercise physiology major with just physiology courses does not meet the core educational information requirements for healthcare professionals. To teach just the physiology of the body without the anatomical facts is to teach essentially half of the body. Such thinking by the administrators and faculty are not acceptable. That is why it is important to initiate a healthy dialogue between what is presently the case and what should be the students' academic reality.

The downward spiral of the traditional anatomy education based on topographical structural anatomy taught by didactic lectures and dissection of the human body remains the most powerful means of presenting and learning anatomy. Both the anatomy class and the use of cadavers must not be dismissed as obsolete. There should be an engaging academic discussion among the department chairs, the university administrators, and the exercise physiologists. The place for teaching functional anatomy in the exercise physiology curricula must be reassessed.

The decrease in the anatomical study of the human body has led to a growing concern. Exercise physiologists, in particular, need more anatomical knowledge, not less. Failing to teach anatomy places the exercise physiologists on the same level as personal trainers (who seem to be strongly interested in stretching the Achilles tendon). However, please note in Box **3** that the Achilles tendon is very thick as it makes contact with the calcaneus. The fact that it can withstand a force of 5000 pounds per square inch without tearing suggests that it does not stretch. Keep in mind, anatomical ignorance has resulted in malpractice suits (Ellis 2002).

The students' education in the anatomical structures of the body is an honor and an obligation. It is also an intimidating task. Under no circumstances should it be replaced by the growing interest in online learning programs or by interactive 3-D animations, regardless of the announcements that the digital format and quick-search DVD facility saves time and/or costs to the department. In fact, while it is unlikely the use of anatomic software will save time when preparing and reviewing lectures (The Conservative Care Specialists 2003), it is clear that students should be provided active hands-on experiences to grasp the integrity of the Achilles tendon to enhance their capacity to prescribe good and safe exercises.

Box 3. The Achilles tendon is a combination of the gastrocnemius and the soleus.

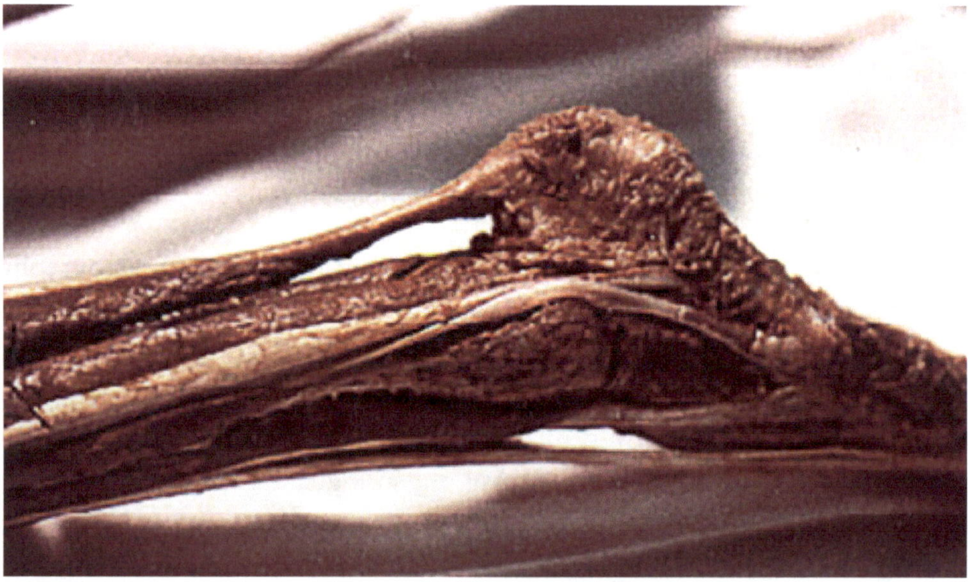

It is important that students use whatever means they have to accept and absorb a new way of thinking about anatomy. The goal is to promote active, life-long learning, and problem solving skills. Whether it is by way of the traditional, lecture-based approach or the hopeful integration of lectures with dissection, the objective is to make a significant and powerful link between both gross anatomy and exercise physiology.

Second, it is essential to the profession of exercise physiologists as healthcare professionals to blend anatomy into the otherwise physiology-driven curriculum. This point brings exercise physiologists back to the question: "Why teach anatomy?" The right answer has to do with safety, expectancy, and ethics along with other considerations that define the academic hierarchy in higher education institutions. It also has to do with exercise medicine of which flexibility exercises represent a means to better health and athletics. Yet, because it is common to do so, time is wasted engaged in the meaningless stretching exercise. With a full integration of an anatomy course and cadaver dissection in the exercise physiology major, students can learn the truth about strength building and range of motion exercises. Otherwise, the failure to engage students in a comprehensive education will continue to marginalize their thinking.

Safety and Effectiveness

For academic exercise physiologists, the human body is the focus of research for publishing purposes. For the non-doctorate exercise physiologists, the profession is about prescribing exercise medicine. Both must have an accurate knowledge of anatomy to ensure the safety of the subjects and clients, respectively. It is therefore a concern that exercise physiologists as college teachers and healthcare entrepreneurs have little to no scientific background in anatomy. This problem of today's decreased anatomical knowledge compared to exercise physiologists decades ago increase the likelihood of leading to safety and effectiveness issues.

Functional anatomy will continue to be the capstone experience of learning the human body. It has survived the most demanding pedagogic test, which is "time" itself. However, as stated earlier, anatomy has been squeezed out of the exercise physiology doctorate curriculum and yet, anatomy is essential for exercise physiologists, especially when they: (a) identify specific exercises to build and maintain the musculoskeletal system; (b) perform cardiovascular assessments and analysis of the client strengths and/or limitations in movement patterns; (c) take the time to explain the human body to clients (Box **4**); and (d) recognize that a referral to a specialist is required.

Box 4. Teaching anatomy, clients, and law suits.

Not only are there educational and professional reasons but also a litigious reason to support the Board Certified Exercise Physiologists' need for anatomical knowledge that is learned by both memorization and visualization. The integration of both stimulates study and increases interest, application, and client safety. Naturally, lectures will remain an important means to teaching applied anatomy. The role of the academic exercise physiologist is to highlight the most important concepts and ideas in an applied and functionally relevant manner.

Students Expect to Learn Anatomy

The students' fascination with anatomy is self-evident. They understand that it is challenging, but it is also rewarding in that they come to understand that part of the body that is seldom analyzed or even talked about. Hence, the students feel it is reasonable to learn anatomy. If asked, the students would say: "We are excited and looking forward to the department's new, state-of-the-art anatomy laboratory that is equipped with cadavers, thus allowing us to observe, dissect, and come to an understanding of the complex architecture of the human body."

Exercise physiology students at the doctorate level are confused when they find out the academic major does not require them to take a course in anatomy. This is a legitimate concern, especially since it impacts the caliber of the students' training. Without a thorough understanding of anatomy with specific implications regarding the client's safety and well-being, disagreements between expectation and reality may inflame future legal claims. Students are at a distinct disadvantage if anatomy is not taught, which is why many students try to teach themselves when it comes to examples where an anatomical specificity is likely to make a difference in a client's safety.

Exercise physiology as a healthcare profession has suffered as a result of its failure to evolve and adapt. Under the old-style doctorate training, students were expected to learn "physiology-oriented" courses with very little understanding of anatomy. Learning just physiology as a rite of passage rather than learning anatomy as well clearly requires significant reform. The teaching of anatomy has suffered because it is regarded as a non-physiology and didactic if not an archaic academic subject. Hence, either the original idea was to reduce the size of the curriculum content by getting rid of anatomy or, perhaps, more simply, get rid of anatomy because the exercise physiologists were not prepared to teach it. Either way, it is an educationally unsound decision that encourages stories of recent graduates who read anatomy books with a weight lifting emphasis without the knowledge necessary to correctly identify the right muscles by name, origin, and insertion.

You Know Anatomy, Right?

Healthcare professionals expect exercise physiologists to have studied anatomy while in college, particularly at the graduate level with the opportunity to dissect cadavers. They are surprised when they learn that anatomy was not a required course in the exercise physiology curriculum, regardless of whether it was at the undergraduate level or the doctorate level. They are even more surprised to learn that the rationale for several decades has been to remove anatomical instruction from the curriculum for more ECG and exercise prescription courses or more strength and conditioning courses. Healthcare professionals are confused as to why the academic exercise physiologists have not included anatomy in the students' list of courses that defines a legitimate exercise physiology major.

The argument not to teach anatomy is a weak perspective, as is the idea to replace the dissecting room and cadavers with more strength and conditioning equipment. Most exercise physiologists have little knowledge of anatomy beyond identifying the biceps brachii, pectoralis major, quadriceps, hamstrings, and the calf muscles. One wonders if they realize just how unprepared they are to work with clients and patients to prevent and treat chronic diseases and disabilities. In fact, the question is this: "As exercise physiologists, do they understand the language of anatomy sufficiently to qualify as a credible healthcare professional when it is necessary to communication anatomical information precisely and effectively" (Box **5**).

Box 5. The anatomy learning center of UCSF.

"Students at UCSF have just begun studies in a new, state-of-the-art anatomy learning center equipped with interactive iPad textbooks, giant video displays and roving cameras that will allow them to observe, discover, and come to understand, in a new way, the complex architecture of the human body."

-- University of California, San Francisco, CA

You can Teach Anatomy, Right?

Anatomy instruction should be part of the doctorate degree. The fact that students do not have access to detailed anatomical lectures and dissection of the body is an unsound decision by academic exercise physiologists who teach at the doctorate level. Also, the lack of access to anatomy is the reason there are few academic exercise physiologists with the academic training and laboratory experience to teach anatomical skills and knowledge? A compelling explanation can be made that they simply do not exist. This is a significant reason why the kinesiology course has been deleted from the curriculum for biomechanics and sports nutrition courses. There seems to be no academic attempt to develop exercise physiology educators with a robust importance in dissected cadaver-based anatomy.

Anatomy is a Required Course

Maybe, in time, it will be clear to academic exercise physiologists and their students to think of anatomy as an integral part of exercise physiology. After all, anatomy should be a required academic course from undergraduate through the doctorate program. When this happens, no doubt there will be some students who may feel that the study of anatomy is a waste of time (Haines *et al.* 2002).

Nonetheless, the students of the profession of exercise physiology should have the opportunity to demonstrate the value of knowing anatomy to their future clients. They should be encouraged to seek out its application, where it is their duty to so. In short, it is a professional defeat in the faculty's responsibility to address with specificity of anatomy in the educational curriculum of exercise physiology. All students of exercise physiology should be taught the same anatomical content and perspective as other healthcare students (*e.g.,* nurses and physical therapists).

Anatomy = Knowledge of Movement

If it is logical to think that academic exercise physiologists would want students to graduate with specific laboratory skills and academic knowledge necessary to help ensure a safe and effective exercise physiology practice, anatomy is a vital part of this knowledge base. While it is not being taught in some academic programs (including medicine), it is possible to reclaim the hands-on anatomy that has produced credible professionals. Even with the technological advances and iPads, there is the need for a thorough lecture-based approach to anatomy. This means that while high-tech visuals are great adjuncts to the teacher's lectures, they are just that – alternatives to the genuine teaching!

Also, while you would not expect exercise physiologists to replace the metabolic cart for actual classroom learning as guided by the teacher, the use of the cart is required for a complete education. Virtual experiences that describe VO_2 max and anatomy are just that – virtual. They are not real interactions between the students, teachers, and cadavers (Box **6**). This point is important, particularly with the emphasis on distance learning, take-home tests, and other technologically driven methods that have taken the place of many teachers.

Box 6. Dissecting cadavers increases students' interest.

Using cadaver dissections to teach anatomy entails active learning with individual effort that substantially increases the students' interest in learning and applying anatomy to clients and patients.

Cadavers = Increased Knowledge

Where students have had the chance to study and dissect cadavers, regardless of the argument of not wanting to touch preserved specimens (Miller *et al.* 2002), more often than otherwise, students take from the experience increased sensitivity for hands-on-laboratory interaction with real world anatomy. The fact is they now get that anatomy is more than the usual view of rote memorization as being a meaningless waste of time. Memorization, in particular, is required to work through a well-planned and effective 3-dimensional view of cadavers (Boone 2001). There are also a variety of other teaching strategies, especially the case-driven inquiry-based analysis and the problem-based group work to learning.

Cadaveric dissection can be among the most profound experiences of the exercise physiology students' education. Synonymous with traditional teaching practices, it is understandable that the majority of the academic institutions favor the use of cadavers to teach anatomy. In addition to dissection aiding in the understanding of the 3-dimensional structure of the human body, dissection allows for increased time spent in studying anatomical variations. Anatomy dissection is an excellent starting point to realizing that muscles and other body parts may (and often do) differ in many ways from the textbook description. Did you know that biceps brachii may occasionally have a third or even a fourth point of origin? This, in return, helps students understand the differences in function as well as pathology.

Anatomy is the Foundation of Function

Why teach anatomy? The palpable answer is because the muscles are the very foundation for human function. To not grasp thoroughly human structure is to set the exercise physiology student up to fail. While this thinking may not be true for all healthcare professions, it is a correct statement for the exercise physiology profession. That is why the Board Certified Exercise Physiologists, as credible healthcare professionals, are required to know the specifics of applied anatomy.

Interestingly, many people with an interest in anatomy are surprised with the findings of Lemons and Griswold (1998). They reported that the nervous system is ranked first followed second by the cardiovascular system. Electrolyte, fluid, and acid-base were ranked third followed by the immune system ranked fourth and, then, in descending rank: the respiratory, endocrine, and musculoskeletal systems. This trend to teach less anatomy and, in particular, to decrease its detail (*e.g.*, origins, insertions, and functions) is an academic, ethical, and potentially a legal problem.

A Way of Thinking

For ~40 years, there has been the continuing discourse of the decreased emphasis in the undergraduate teaching of anatomy. Yet, it is very clear that anatomy is practical and functional. Otherwise, how would an exercise physiologist know the "why" and "why not" to perform certain strength building exercises with muscle-specific insight? How about range of motion exercises? Learning anatomy is critical when teaching flexibility exercises. It is difficult to calculate the serious problems that result from trainers and others without a knowledge of anatomy. Teaching the principles of anatomy is more than the identification of osteological landmarks, joint actions, and memorizing the origins and insertions of muscles, especially if the students do not understand the concept of biological variation among clients and/or patients.

While it is important that college teachers do not forget to teach the names of anatomical structures, they must place greater emphasis on the "language of anatomy". In other words, exercise physiologists must have the ability to reason (*i.e.*, to see with the mind's eye) the relationships of individual muscles to each other. This is done by recalling images in a 3-dimensional display of actual shape and purpose (Boone 1990), which is rich with anatomical information.

When anatomy is taught as a language of function based on anatomical structure, assimilation of core knowledge and student understanding are possible. The challenge then should not be to diminish the teaching of anatomy, but rather to maximize the learning benefit that results from the appropriate use of dissection and other teaching resources. For certain, failing to teach the musculoskeletal system is not the answer. How else are exercise physiologists going to absorb the link between dysfunction and atypical structure that results from chronic diseases, muscle tendon traumas, or disabilities? Here, the study of anatomy requires a thorough understanding of origins, insertions, and specific osteological terms.

Hardly enough can be said about the language of anatomy. It entails the ability to explain the engagement of specific muscles across a joint(s) and why. For example, to perform a chin up on the high bar requires the arms to undergo either extension or adduction at the shoulder joints while the elbow joints are flexing. There are 10 muscles that are responsible for shoulder adduction: latissimus dorsiteres major, teres minor, infraspinatus, posterior deltoid, long head of triceps brachii, subscapularis, short head of biceps brachii, coracobrachialis, and sternal fibers of the pectoralis major. For these muscles to respond appropriately at the shoulder joint, the scapular must undergo retraction and downward rotation. There are four muscles responsible for this action: levator scapulae, rhomboid minor, rhomboid major, and pectoralis minor. At the elbow joint, flexion is carried out by eight muscles: biceps brachii, brachialis, brachioradialis, pronator teres, flexor carpi radialis, palmaris longus, flexor carpi ulnaris, and flexor digitorum superficialis. All 22 skeletal muscles are used to control the return to the original position.

Often, what is not recognized in the list of muscles in the individual osteological connections to the skeletal system and, therefore, their functional relationship to each other relative to a particular joint. As an example, what is the right answer to the following questions?

- Which muscle inserts under the shoulder joint by way of the medial lip of the bicipital groove?
- What muscle inserts essentially in the same place but superior to the muscle that arises in part from the dorsal spine of T6?
- Two muscles are often referred to as one muscle, given their insertion point. Do these muscles arise from the anterior or dorsal surface of the scapula?

- The spine of the scapula ends in a process that articulates with the distal end of the clavicle. Both bones allow for the origin of two functional parts of a muscle. The part arising from the spine is referred to as the _____ muscle.
- The inferior aspect of the glenoid fossa gives rise to a muscle that inserts on the ulna. What is the name of the muscle?

While the list of questions is essentially endless, the point of the exercise is this. The correct answer to the questions is the first, five muscles in the order indicated above that produce shoulder adduction. What is not so obvious is that the answer to each question is a function of having knowledge of the origins, insertions, and actions of the specific muscles and how they relate to each other. As a further example, given that there are eight elbow flexors, the question might be how many nerves are responsible for that action? The answer is "four". Which nerve then is all powerful and which is least important? The answer is as follows: The musculocutaneous nerve to the biceps brachii and brachialis muscles, and the ulnar nerve to the flexor carpi ulnaris.

Final Thoughts

The final question is this: Would you take your car to a mechanic who does not know where all the parts of the engine are located, much less what each part does? Of course, the answer is "No". So, if you are an academic exercise physiologist, why would you allow your students to graduate without an adequate anatomical preparation to professionally and safely work as an exercise physiologist? There is absolutely no doubt that a non-doctorate exercise physiologist needs a thorough grounding in the principles, concepts, and language of anatomy (Box **7**). The use of didactic lectures along with cadaver-based dissection opportunities, problem-based workshops, computer programs, plastic models, and other teaching tools are indispensable in teaching, comprehending and successfully learning the principles of anatomy.

Box 7. The language of anatomy.

Strangely enough, there is not even a perception among exercise physiologists that the depth of anatomical knowledge of their students is inadequate. Where is the unease among exercise physiologists and the general public? The language of anatomy should be taught to the students so that they can effectively communicate with their clients and patients.

GLOSSORY

Academic preparation	Identification of the right academic setting and courses in a student's education.
Hands-on dissection	Direct personal contact and attention to dissection.
Language of anatomy	Terms that define and characterize anatomical positions and parts.
Meaningless stretching	Waste of time performing exercises that fail to stretch intended muscles.
Science of physiology	Intellectual activity encompassing the systematic study of the branch of biology that deals with the functions.

REFERENCES

Boone, T (1990) Imagery and teaching: some reflections. *J Phys Educ, Recreat Dance,* 62, 45-9. [http://dx.doi.org/10.1080/07303084.1990.10604579]

Boone, T (2001) Anatomy: the forgotten piece of the beginning. *Professionalization of Exercise Physiologyonline,* 4 [Online], http://www.css.edu/users/tboone2/asep/ANATOMYandExercisePhysiologists.html

Ellis, H (2002) Medico-legal and its links with surgical anatomy. *Surgery,* 20, 1-2.

Haines, DE, Hutchins, JB & Lynch, JC (2002) Medical neurobiology: do we teach neurobiology in a format that is relevant to the clinical setting? *Anat Rec,* 269, 99-106. [http://dx.doi.org/10.1002/ar.10073] [PMID: 12001216]

Lemons, DE & Griswold, JG (1998) Defining the boundaries of physiological understanding: the benchmarks curriculum model. *Am J Physiol,* 275, S35-45. [PMID: 16161224]

Miller, SA, Perrotti, W, Silverthorn, DU, Dalley, AF & Rarey, KE (2002) From college to clinic: reasoning over memorization is key for understanding anatomy. *Anat Rec,* 269, 69-80. [http://dx.doi.org/10.1002/ar.10071] [PMID: 12001213]

Paalman, MH (2000) Why teach anatomy? Anatomists respond. *Anat Rec,* 261, 1-2. [http://dx.doi.org/10.1002/(SICI)1097-0185(20000215)261:1<1::AID-AR1>3.0.CO;2-3] [PMID: 10700728]

Reidenberg, JS & Laitman, JT (2002) The new face of gross anatomy. *Anat Rec,* 269, 81-8. [http://dx.doi.org/10.1002/ar.10076] [PMID: 12001214]

The Conservative Care Specialists Interactive functional anatomy – DVD. [Online], http://www.optp.com

CHAPTER 5

Teaching Anatomy to Exercise Physiology Students

Abstract: "The taboo against desecrating the bodies of the dead goes back many centuries; it was prohibited by both ancient Greek and Roman religions. Cadaver dissection is essential for the acquisition of anatomical language. The first recorded instance of medical dissection of human bodies is in the sixth century BCE, when the Greek philosopher Alcmaeon began his research. In 275 BCE, Herophilus of Chalcedon founded the first school of anatomy at the Museum of Alexandria, in part to encourage his students to overcome their fear of dissecting human bodies" (http://knarf.english.upenn.edu/Contexts/dissect.html). Given the significance of this quote, students, teachers, researchers, and surgeons are still asking questions: Is dissection the *only* way to learn anatomy? Why don't they have cadavers to dissect? When teaching anatomy, which is best – cadavers or computers? Can the YouTube help students learn anatomy? Is it better than dissection? Do students have sufficient knowledge of clinical anatomy with just lectures?

Keywords: Anatomic software, ASEP, Exercise medicine, Medical dissection.

INTRODUCTION

Teaching the principles of cadaver dissection is an important part of the history of medicine. The first recorded dissection was around 300 B.C. by Herophilus. He is known as the father of anatomy. In the school of Alexandria, the use of anatomic dissection was the primary method of learning anatomy. During the 14th and 15th centuries, French and Italian professors used cadavers to teach anatomy. After that, only a few cadavers were dissected until the 17th and 18th centuries (Korf & Wicht 2004). The first medical school in United States was founded in 1765 at the College of Philadelphia. In 1767 and 1782, additional medical programs were created in New York and Boston, respectively. Michelangelo and Leonardo da

Tommy Boone

Vinci carried out dissection to enhance their artistic work (Dyer & Thorndike 2000).

Before dissection became legal, anatomy schools relied on grave robbers to obtain cadavers. Some bodies were illegally circulated to other countries. In 1831, the Anatomical Act of Massachusetts was passed. It allowed medical schools to receive unclaimed cadavers. The Act moved cadavers into the laboratory setting (Stimec *et al.* 2010). Additional legislation resulted in better controls that brought anatomy education into hospitals and colleges. The body donation program was gradually accepted. Cadavers were regarded as scientific assets.

In 1882, the College of Physicians and Surgeons of Chicago offered a three-year curriculum that included the dissection of cadavers. Because anatomic material was difficult to obtain, the Anatomical Gift Association of Illinois was founded in Chicago in 1968 with the aim to legally embalm and disperse cadavers throughout the state, using deeds signed over by soon-to-be donors. Deed-based programs now exist in all states except Wyoming. Today, the Anatomy Gift Act produces cadavers every year for medical education and research.

Aside from the *Body-Worlds* that exhibits anatomical art of phenomenal dissections and plastinations created by Gunther Von Hagens in Germany in 1978, anatomists are still very much interested in cadavers. They understand that the plastinated bodies and body parts along with the anatomical software, and other imaging methods are increasingly being used to teach and do research. But, once again, their interest is in anatomy taught by cadaveric dissection, prosection, and other anatomical materials (and the functional dynamics of bones) (Box **1**).

It is important that interest in cadaver dissection be sustained not only to benefit members of the healthcare professions, but to help ensure that the professionals thoroughly understand anatomy and its application to healthcare diseases and disabilities. Removing cadavers from the academic setting is likely to cause a major shift in a time-honored tradition, which in turn will have a negative effect on anatomy education. Cadavers allow students to gain unique insights into human body, which have thus far (for the most part) been reserved for a select few medical professionals at best (Box **2**).

Box 1. The osteology of a gymnastics dismount.

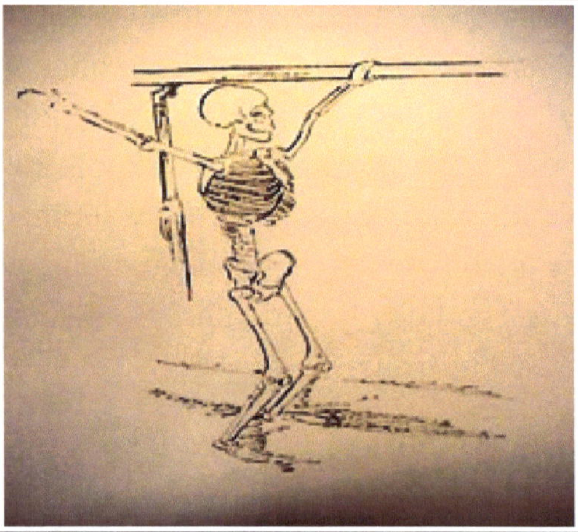

The upper and lower limbs are characterized by their mobility and ability to grasp and conduct motor skills, such as dismounting from the parallel bars in men's gymnastics. Note the grasp of the left hand on the bar, which is made possible primarily by the muscles of the anterior forearm. The knee flexion is controlled by the anterior thigh muscles (known as the quadriceps femoris) that insert on the tibia tuberosity. The dorsi-flexion of the ankle joint is controlled by the plantar flexors (6 from the posterior side of the leg and 2 from the lateral side of the leg).

Box 2. Why is dissection important?

"Dissection of the human body is the only method of direct observation and measurement of the structures, organs, bones, ligaments and tendons that allow the body to function. Direct dissection is a fundamental part of the training of physicians and other care providers. Physicians cannot treat disease or trauma without a complete understanding of anatomy."

--Anatomical Gift Association of Illinois 2016

Changes in exercise physiology such as using cadavers in addition to other laboratory functions enhance the core curriculum and increase the importance placed on learning through dissection. The ASEP leaders maintain that a in-depth appreciation of anatomy by cadaver dissections should be part of every exercise physiologist's academic major.

Anatomy in Exercise Physiology

When students undergo cadaver-based learning by dissecting cadavers, their ability to conceptualize anatomical structures is significantly better than without the hands-on experience. The dissection experience itself is awesome. It provides students with the actual thickness of muscles, how they are oriented to each other, as well as the layering of muscles. They can see and touch the origins, insertions, and nerves that go to the muscles, thus help to understand specific functions.

In fact, as Chair of the Department of Exercise Physiology, it was obvious that the students wanted access to cadaver dissection. That is part of the reason why I created the Anatomy Laboratory with cadavers. The hands-on experience was packed with clinically relevant anatomical talk, facts, and active learning that aided the necessary memorization.

The disadvantage in using cadavers centered primarily on the cost, which varied at the time from \$2,000 to \$4,000 each. There was also an upfront cost for a ventilation system in the cadaver laboratory. The student laboratory fees helped. Most of the time, students were assessed a \$100 lab fee. There were ~12 to 15 graduate students per year and four cadavers per year. With transportation cost and other experiences, the overall cost was ~\$10,000 per academic year. When the department budget is not set up to cover the cost, it may be possible to request sharing expenses and laboratory time with other departments (*e.g.,* physical therapy and/or occupational therapy).

Some judge that the color, smell, and texture of cadavers are sufficiently different from actual life that the laboratory expenses and time in preparation and dissection are wasted. They argue that anatomical pictures in textbooks are just as good if not better. Well, frankly, such an argument is inaccurate. Even the use of 3-dimensional images and structures is not equal to studying the actual muscles and other structures of a cadaver (Box **3**).

Box 3. The lack of anatomy is self-evident.

It is most unfortunate but true that exercise physiologists in the United States have continued to demonstrate deficiencies in the knowledge of anatomy, which is a critical foundation to understanding human movement and treatment protocols. Fortunately, the students of exercise physiology who were exposed to cadaver dissection and who are going on to get the doctorate degree will likely help in providing cadaver opportunities to their students. Teaching the principles of anatomy within the dissecting laboratory introduces students to the reality of hands-on visualization, the concept of biological variation in points of origin and insertion. The art and science of teaching weight lifting and flexibility will be improved.

Presently, a small number of exercise physiology programs teach anatomy. This is a huge difference from 40 to 50 years ago when anatomy was taught in a kinesiology course. Initially, students of physical education were expected to know the origins and insertions of the major muscles. During the 1970s and 1980s many of the academic majors were changed to kinesiology, exercise science, human performance, or one of a dozen similar names (Boone 2001).

In America, the academic degree title is confusing and misleading due to the academic exercise physiologists turning a blind eye to the students' problems at the undergraduate level. After all, they believe that they are "physiologists" and not "exercise physiologists". Their logic makes no sense at all and yet, it is part of the many reasons why the teaching of human anatomy to the students of exercise physiology is problematic. Unfortunately, they have failed in leading the transition of exercise physiology from its original physical education connection into their existence, perhaps, due to the sports medicine link (Box **4**).

Box 4. The failure of academic exercise physiologists.

It is well-known that as the population ages, the prevalence and costs of bone and joint diseases are only going to increase. Therefore, now more than ever before, knowledge of musculoskeletal anatomy is imperative in exercise physiology. But, presently, the exercise physiologist's lack of anatomical knowledge and clinical experience is a failure to support professionalism in exercise physiology. The exercise physiologists' dedication to a cognitive mastery of musculoskeletal concepts and treatment using exercise as the primary prescriptive form of medicine is a necessity.

While the influence of sports medicine on exercise physiology has been explored in articles published in the ASEP professionalism journal, *Professionalization of Exercise Physiology-online*, exercise physiologists still comprehend very little about how or why students should learn anatomy (Boone 2001; Boone 2003). To make matters worse, academic exercise physiologists are not discussing the need to teach anatomy. Moreover, they are not adding anatomy to the students' list of courses. Also, you can forget about the students' exposure to cadavers, prosected and/or plastinated specimens, lectures, tutorials, web-based, and/or computer-based resources.

No one is asking the question: "Why is it that exercise physiologists do not know anatomy?" Part of the answer is this: The literature on exercise physiology is influenced by human performance and strength training research. There is also the view that anatomy is all about memorization and reciting information as though that does not happen in the exercise physiology course.

Yet, the ability to remember, visualize, and problem solve anatomic structures is important to the success of healthcare professionals. They also need a mind-body understanding of the human body (Boone 2010). This is why I created the first-ever psychophysiology course for exercise physiology students at the University of Southern Mississippi in Hattiesburg, MS in the mid-1980s and later at The College of Saint Scholastica in Duluth, MN in the mid-1990s.

Unless anatomy becomes a regular course in the curriculum, the healthcare practice of exercise physiologists cannot be complete. Thus, it is clear that exercise physiologists must get their minds around the following questions: Firstly, what is the language of teaching anatomy and how best can it be taught? Secondly, why is it important that exercise physiologists know anatomy and physiology? For certain, exercise physiologists who want to work with clients who have musculoskeletal disabilities or who want to develop their muscle strength and/or endurance need a strong background in anatomy. Whether anatomy should be taught as a lecture only course or as a lecture plus cadaver dissection remains to be analyzed by the profession.

Should the study of anatomy not require cadaver dissection, it will no doubt be a major mistake. This point of view is no different from the emphasis placed on exercise physiology concepts without having a metabolic cart, bicycle ergometer, or other laboratory equipment. The scope of exercise physiology goes beyond the emphasis on just physiology. Hence, if its healthcare practitioners are to acquire the knowledge necessary to promote the "good" of the client, they must achieve a more engaging view of the exercise physiologists' role in healthcare. This means avoiding the mindset that encourages an over-dependence on physiology (Box **5**).

Box 5. A strong background in anatomy increases safety in weight lifting.

Without a strong anatomical foundation, it is next to impossible to teach students how to use the correct weight lifting exercises properly and to safely address certain clinical scenarios. In short, the point is that even years of working out with weights do not allow for an expert opinion in regards to all subjects and especially the health challenged populations. Far too often so-called experts produce a simplistic and distorted view of resistance training. Quality healthcare is a direct dialogue between the client/patient and healthcare professional. Therefore, if students just lift weights with knowing anatomy, they will not develop the requisite reasoning of being a professional.

Where educational institutions focus their time on securing student tuition dollars, new curriculum ideas and straight thinking regarding professionalism are often at the end of the list of concerns. This is a problem just as the lack of anatomy in exercise physiology is a problem. Both have triggered the need for change which, in turn, means that a higher academic standard in exercise physiology is required, as suggested by the American Society of Exercise Physiologists (ASEP 2007).

Members of the ASEP Board of Directors recognize that the students of exercise physiology need a rigorous and complete academic education to safely care for their clients and/or patients. Thus, it is academically a mistake for exercise physiology students to continue taking the same science courses as physical education majors. Clearly, "physiology" is at the center of "exercise physiology" but is the study exercise biomechanics and sports, rehabilitation of lifestyle diseases, exercise nutrition, psychophysiology of health and exercise, spirituality and well-being, and, yes, anatomy (Box **6**) if the students are going to be prepared to practice exercise physiology.

Box 6. Where is the anatomy dissection?

"Computer models, study modules, problem-based workshops, and computer-based tutorials are filling the classrooms at medical schools" (Older 2004). These new trends have changed the role of dissection in teaching anatomy. Ask yourself, "Where is the anatomy dissection?" Anatomy dissection is important, isn't it? Yet, unfortunately, there is the perception among many exercise physiologists that anatomy is an unnecessary expense and waste of time. Why, then, is biomechanics more important than anatomy? If it isn't, where is the debate? Why aren't exercise physiologists promoting the ASEP 21st century view of the profession *vs.* the 20th century exercise science perspective?

The ASEP leaders believe that the teaching of anatomy is an essential course in the exercise physiology curriculum (Box **7**). Traditional anatomical knowledge is too important to the Board Certified Exercise Physiologists not to teach it. Once again, as has been mentioned, since there are only a few doctorate programs in exercise physiology in the United States that students can dissect cadavers, it is important to start thinking differently about anatomy.

Combining kinesiology (*i.e.,* anatomy) with sports biomechanics is a problem. There is no way anatomy can be learned without engaging students in lectures and laboratory experiences dedicated to the study of anatomy. Frankly, a year of anatomy would be much better for an exercise physiologist than a year of studying macromolecules. Yet, molecular biology is viewed more important than either anatomy instruction or cadaver dissection.

Box 7. Prescribing exercise medicine safely requires knowing anatomy.

A key component to all change is a vision that is compelling, lifting, and to the point. The ASEP leaders believe their vision is rooted in the core purpose to help students, to help the profession, and to help society. Exercise physiology students of today need to learn more than the students who graduated 10 years ago. The exercise physiology practice has changed especially over the past decade, and rapid change continues today. The emergence of "exercise as medicine" requires that the graduates are advanced in their understanding and application of exercise medicine in health, disease, and athletics.

The solution is not the random about-face to an atlas of anatomy. It is scarcely enough to permit a comprehensive analysis of the anatomy. Students need to undertake the study of muscles just as they are required to engage other laboratory experiences, especially the skills that undergird physiology and exercise testing. Each course involves specific processing of information, cooperation among the students and teachers, and verbal discussion before their peers as to what they know and do not know. The subject matter must be taught in a mixed fashion to avoid fragmentation. Professionalism and standards of practice must be part of the exercise physiology course work and not simply reduced to a one-time lecture or discussion (ASEP 2016).

The hands-on approach to learning anatomy, particularly through the use of cadaveric dissection, is the logical means to absorbing and learning anatomy. Dissecting and individualizing the learning process is vital to the future practice of exercise physiology. In fact, it increases the prospect of professional success as healthcare practitioners. But, to begin with, there must be the opportunity to study anatomy in the accredited curriculum for exercise physiologists. Second, there must be exercise physiologists who know anatomy and who know how to teach cadaver dissection. Third, exercise physiologists must remove themselves from the narrowed interest of – *physiology only* – that co-occur with the research interests of the 20th century exercise physiologists (Box **8**).

Box 8. ASEP leaders are speaking the truth.

"The best way to speak the truth is to know it clearly, believe it implicitly, love it sincerely, live it courageously, and proclaim it zealously."

-- Clifton J. Allen

Final Thoughts

However appropriate it is, as an academic course in exercise physiology, sports biomechanics is an inadequate substitution for the study of anatomy. One of the most interesting concepts in athletics and health is biological variation. The fact that no two athletes are exactly the same anatomically deserves discussion and analysis. Understanding muscle variations, whether it is the origin, insertion, or both is very useful in developing individualized exercise prescriptions.

Today's undergraduates should not simply be dismissed as fitness instructors or personal trainers. The current ASEP trend and vision of Board Certified Exercise Physiologists as healthcare professionals requires that the students are prepared for unpredictable variations in human anatomy just as they are expected to know electrocardiography when it comes to working with post-myocardial infarction patients in cardiac rehabilitation (Box **9**). Unfortunately, one of the consequences of a poor undergraduate education is the failure to act appropriately with clients and/or patients. The actual study of anatomy will help correct this problem.

Box 9. Medical schools turn a blind eye to teaching anatomy.

"Medical students have been taught anatomy in the same way since medieval times - by dissection of human cadavers. In medical schools around the country, however, the emphasis has now shifted from students dissecting to demonstrator led teaching. The origins and insertions are out of favor, and the clinical relevance of the anatomy we learn is in favor. Having completed my preclinical studies, I ask myself whether the changes in the style of teaching are for the better or have gone too far. My experience of the teaching of anatomy is a poor one. Instead of actively participating in dissections, up to 11 students gather around prepared prosections and are taught by a demonstrator, which takes the fun out of learning anatomy. The hands on approach must be a more effective way of learning anatomy than trying to absorb information passively from a demonstration."

-- Afzal Mohammed (2000)

The ASEP leadership is convinced that a new day is dawning for the profession of exercise physiology. As Dr. Harvey said in his 1931 book, "Change is constant. It is going on. It will go on." In time, anatomy will again be part of the exercise physiology list of required courses (Box **10**). Perhaps, each of us will discover in ourselves a sense of purpose that will help align anatomy with physiology. Such a purpose makes good sense. Why not create a vision and a commitment to the expectation that all exercise physiology students will have the opportunity to study anatomy. A vision of this kind can be the force to make a profound difference in the students' education. And, frankly, as W. Somerset Maugham wrote of a lecturer advising first-year medical students, "You will have to learn many tedious things which you will forget the moment you have passed your final examination, but in anatomy it is better to have learned and lost than never to have learned at all."

Box 10. Time requires change, but the right kind.

"Change is constant. It is going on. It will go on. We do not know what we shall be, but in light of our past we must expect the age-long progress to continue."

- B. C. H. Harvey, MD (1931)

GLOSSORY

Anatomic software	Software for learning, reviewing, and teaching anatomy.
ASEP	American Society of Exercise Physiologists is the professional organization of exercise physiologists.
Exercise medicine	A branch of exercise physiology that deals with the prescription of exercise in the prevention and treatment of chronic diseases and disabilities.
Medical dissection	Process of cutting apart or separating tissue as, for example, in the study of anatomy.

REFERENCES

American Society of Exercise Physiologists. ASEP vision, [Online], http://www.asep.org/ organization.

American Society of Exercise Physiologists ASEP standards of practice. [Online], https://www.asep.org/index.php/organization/ practice/.

Anatomical Gift Association of Illinois, Why is dissection important?. [Online], http://www.agaillinois.org/dispo.htm.

Boone, T (2001) Anatomy: the forgotten piece of the beginning *Professionalization of Exercise*

Physiologyonline, 4 [Online], http://faculty.css.edu/tboone2/asep/ANATOMYandExercisePhysiologists.html.

Boone, T (2003) Why teach anatomy *Professionalization of Exercise Physiologyonline,* 6:3 [Online], http://faculty.css.edu/tboone2/asep/WhyTeachAnatomy.html.

Boone, T (2010) Integrating spirituality and exercise physiology: toward a new understanding of health. The Edwin Mellen Press, Lewiston, New York.

Dyer, GS & Thorndike, ME (2000) Quidne mortui vivos docent? The evolving purpose of human dissection in medical education. *Acad Med,* 75, 969-79.
[http://dx.doi.org/10.1097/00001888-200010000-00008] [PMID: 11031139]

Harvey, BC (1931) *Simple lessons in human anatomy.* American Medical Association, Chicago, Illinois.

Korf, HW & Wicht, H (2004) The public cadaver. *Nature,* 428, 805.
[http://dx.doi.org/10.1038/428805a] [PMID: 15103356]

Mohammed, A (2000) Teaching anatomy must change. *Student BMJ,* 8, 1-44. [February.].

Older, J (2004) Anatomy: a must for teaching the next generation *Surgeon,* 2, 79-90. [Online]. http://www.rcsed.ac.uk/journal/svol2_2/20200003.html.

Stimec, BV, Draskic, M & Fasel, JH (2010) Cadaver procurement for anatomy teaching: legislative challenges in a transition-related environment. *Med Sci Law,* 50, 45-9.
[http://dx.doi.org/10.1258/msl.2009.009008] [PMID: 20349695]

CHAPTER 6

Use of Imagery in Anatomy

Abstract: Teachers must acknowledge that rote memorization is rather useless when students are not encouraged to visualize the structures. There is a huge volume of detail and integrated content when anatomy is blended with mental pictures. The mind can be taught to scan the origins, insertions, and functions of muscles just as computers can scan and create three-dimensional pictures. The brain does not know the difference between what is real and what is not real. Thus, when you visualize (*i.e.,* see with the mind's eye) the latissimus dorsi muscle and its origin and insertion, the electrical signals of the thinking-visualization process are essentially the same as seeing it on a cadaver.

Keywords: Blink transformations, Creating images, Image rotation, Imagery, Mental scanning, Stored information, Verbalizers, Visualizers.

INTRODUCTION

The mental image is one of the oldest, left alone issues in intellectual science. It is so misunderstood that psychologists have both maintained and rejected its existence, even though it has always been with us. Few would dispute the ability to produce a mental image. Everyone generates images and, yet evidently, many professionals disagree on what is an image. To mull over what is an image is to ask questions without an obvious answer. Few people feel comfortable speaking about a topic when there is little agreement (Boone 2001).

About all a person can say is that a mental image appears to resemble the experience of seeing an object that is not actually present. Controversy, neglect, and speculation provide little support in understanding the "experience of seeing" a mental image. How a mental image (or mental visualization) helps with the learning of anatomy is not easily explained. Yet, anatomy teachers argue that

Tommy Boone

creating a mental image of the pectoralis major is helpful in understanding its functions. As an example, close your eyes and "see with your mind's eye" the clavicular part of the anterior chest muscle as it helps to flex the shoulder joint.

Critics disagree by asking, "How is it possible to see an object and then rotate it?" Hence, the question: Does the brain create mental pictures? If so, what are the specifics for defining a mental picture and, equally important, what types of information does the picture provide? Finding an answer to these questions is not easy even among the best of psychologists and exercise physiologists.

Recalling an Image

If human mental imagery exists, can we be taught to recall specific images? Is the neural status of an image based on memorization and/or visualization? Or, is it simply a function of the memory process? If we can recover and reconstruct information at will, we can learn to modify it. That is, if a student is asked to imagine the quadriceps and assuming the student sees the quadriceps in his or her mind's eye, can the student recall images of functional association (such as hip flexion and/or knee extension by specific muscles) (Box **1**)?

Box 1. The anterior thigh muscles.

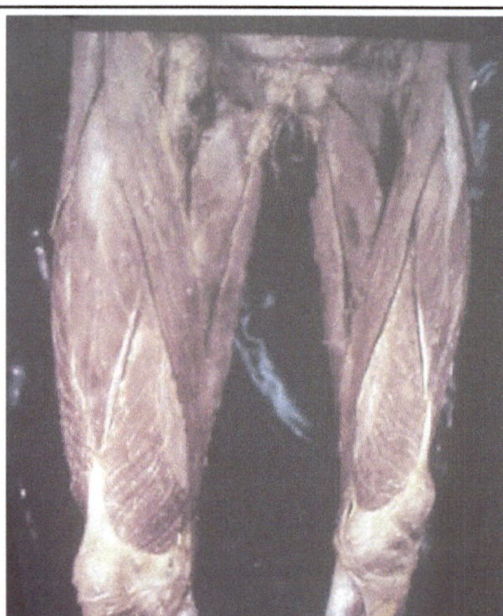

Take a moment and look at the picture of the muscles of the thigh. Do you see the vastus medialis, rectus femoris, and the vastus lateralis? Understandably, you cannot see the vastus intermedius. But, you can imagine "seeing" it as well as the points of origin for each of the four muscles. One of the muscles originates from across the hip, which is the rectus femoris (specifically, its origin is the anterior inferior iliac spine). Imagine the greater trochanter and lateral lip of the linea aspera and you will have the origin of the vastus lateralis, which inserts *via* common quadriceps tendon. Note the muscle cross the thigh from the hip region to the medial side of the knee joint. This is the sartorius muscle. It arises from the ASIS to flex the thigh and inserts *via* the proximal anterior medial aspect of the tibia. It works with the gracilis to flex the knee joint.

The idea of seeing the knee extensors with image vividness is first linked to specific information acquired from an instructor or an anatomy book. The mental image of the quadriceps is not like looking at a picture in a book or even the quadriceps of another person. Instead, one would conclude that the quadriceps is a visualized construction that is considered a rough copy of the actual muscles. The muscles exist as an image that takes a lot of practice in visualization to see the small details that are obvious only after a disciplined approach to creating images. For example, the image of the short head of the biceps brachii at the shoulder joint is better in the person who works at creating images.

To assert further that mental images do exist, take a moment to picture a car but not just any car. Picture a black Ford truck and then a yellow Ford truck. Very likely, you were able to pictured a Ford truck and, if so, a black Ford truck and then a yellow one. This means you created the image in your mind's eye. Now, picture the same truck in red. It should be clear that images exist regardless of the fact that it is hard to explain or define them.

What is important is when a person visualizes something, such as the quadriceps muscles, the image is specific to the thighs of the lower limbs. Now, to further demonstrate this point, when the same person is asked to visualize the vastus medialis muscle, the image is that of what one would see in the anatomy picture of the quadriceps. The image may be taken from a stored memory of a textbook picture or an anatomy dissection at some point in one's past. With practice, there isn't much difference between the textbook and what one sees by way of a mental picture.

Think about volleyball, soccer, and baseball. With the recalling back of a sport, the mind creates mental images consistent with known or stored information specific to each athlete. This is not to downplay the role of language in generating thoughts and/or ideas, but rather to highlight the part that visual thinking plays in recalling information. Visual thinking plays a vital role in recall and memory of facts. Again, as an example, visualize a motorcycle and now visualize a bicycle. In less than seconds, the stockpile of information explains the differences between the two. It is also true with learning anatomy or the multi-factors of life in general.

Remember the brain does not know the difference between what is real and what is not real. Thus, when you visualize the latissimus dorsi muscle and its origins and insertion, the electrical signals of the thinking-visualization process are the same as seeing it on a cadaver.

Visualizing Depth

What is also revealing in the images is the fact that they are either two- or three-dimensional. A person can visualize a truck from the driver's side or the back seat and see only the top or the front of the truck or any of a number of different views. Or, a person may decide to look at the truck by seeing through it, for example, back to front and appreciate that it has a third dimension referred to as depth. Thus, a person's memory representation is extremely helpful in recalling information that is subject to intentional representation that is depended on the information that is requested. For example, if the intention is to visualize the shoulder flexors that arise in part from the scapula, the process of looking at and transforming images undergoes at least three steps:

1. **Image generation** (mentally picturing or "seeing" the shoulder region and muscles);
2. **Image inspection** (also called "scanning" specifically to visually locate the shoulder flexors); and
3. **Image transformation** (mentally identifying specific muscles that flex the shoulder joint).

In regards to anatomy, the process of seeing, scanning, and transforming images encourages the recall of anatomical facts and information specific to the functions of muscles. As an example, to mentally picture the axillary nerve to the deltoid muscles, you may begin by "seeing" the anterior shoulder region. To "scan" the region, you would visually locate the axillary nerve arising from the posterior cord of the brachial plexus. Note that the nerve passes dorsal to the proximal end of the humerus to innervate the deltoid muscles from underneath the humerus. Now, rotate the image and look at it from the posterior side. Release the posterior and middle deltoid muscles from the spine and acromion process of the scapula, respectively. Note that with moving the deltoid laterally, the axillary nerve can be seen. If necessary, transform the image by either enlarging it or by rotating it. By zooming in on the nerve, it is a simple matter of making the image larger. Moving back from the image is the essence of making it smaller, perhaps to see all of the nerves that comprise the brachial plexus (just beneath the distal end of the clavicle). The rotation of images allows for anatomical information that might otherwise not be intuitively obvious, but exists nevertheless.

Create a mental image of your apartment or parents' home. "See" with your mind's eye the physical design as though you were standing at the front door. Notice how everything is part of the image. For example, note whether there are steps that leading up to the front door, the type of door, the size of the door, the number of windows, and how the windows are framed. Everything is in the image. Now, allow your mind's eye to rotate the image that represents the front door and the front of the house. Rotate the image to your left and then to the right. Notice that you can see exactly what your mind creates. The rotation of the image that characterizes the house is possible in considerable detail in every direction. It is without question an image of multi-dimensions (Box **2**).

Box 2. The link between perception and intelligence.

"The evolution of images is a kind of intermediate between that of the perceptions and that of the intelligence." -- Jean Piaget

To further promote the power of images, try allowing yourself to be part of the image by visualizing yourself inside, for example, your bedroom prior to leaving for college. Relax and allow the image to develop. What do you see? Your eyes may remain open or close. Do you see your chair? What is the shape? Is it small or large? What color is the chair? Is it made of metal or wood? Is there a picture on the wall behind the desk? Is there a window? Is there a desk in the room? How many pieces of furniture are in the room? How many doors lead from the room? Where do they go? Now, allow your mind to see the inside of your parents' home all at once. How many rooms, bathrooms, and bedrooms are there? Is the dwelling one or more floors made of bricks or wood?

Have you notice that answers to the questions correspond closely with the actual structure and furniture in the dwelling. The structures of the human body can be remembered by creating the same kind of mental images that allow for storage of important anatomical and physiological bits of information. It is as easy as the reconstruction of actual perceptual experiences from the anatomy laboratory or from drawings the teacher placed on the chalkboard.

Blink Transformations

Artists, instructors, and students who use visual thinking will also use "blink transformations" in which an image is allowed to fade (such as the brachialis muscle) while being replaced by a new, different image in its place (perhaps, the biceps brachii). Blink transformations are also used in a variety of sports, including gymnastics when a coach closes his eyes momentarily to see a new image of a skill at a new location, position, or size in the specific routine. The new image encourages the recall of specific information that might not be readily available with the first or second image. It also allows for a mental image to compare the execution of the skill with the desired execution.

The new image that is created by blink transformation is helpful in recalling facts specific to well defined issues. For example, take the view of different areas of the right scapula. Visualize the dorsal view of the right scapula either positioned on the dorsal surface of the thorax of a person standing in front of you or at a few feet in front of your mind's eyes as a separate, stand alone bone. Note that the dorsal surface of the image approximates the dorsal view of the scapula if you were looking at it in an anatomy book. Move your view of the image to the dorsal spine that begins at the base of the spine (which is located about one-third way down from the tip of the superior angle on the medial side of the scapula). Now, follow the visual path of the spine laterally to the acromion process that is located superior to the glenoid cavity.

Close your eyes and see the scapula by itself. It is now three to four times its normal size. It is located in front of your eyes. Open your eyes and image the scapula once again. Look at the superior angle at the top left, medial margin of the right scapula. Contrast the osteological site with the inferior angle as the lowest tip of the scapula. Note that the two angles are created by borders. The superior border of the scapula and the medial border create the superior angle while the lateral border and the medial border create the inferior angle (Boone 1990).

Now, try this mental image experiment. Create an image of the door to your office or apartment (Box **3**). On which side is it hinged? Does your office or apartment have windows and, if so, how many windows are there? Answering these questions begin by imagining the door and the windows by using blink transformations. Likewise, create a mental image of the desk in your office or "see" bed and/or bathroom. Where is the desk located in the room? What are the items positioned close to the desk, and what is on top of the desk? Answers to these questions are a function of the mind creating images from stored information that associates with the images in exactly the same way we understand the various osteological sites of the scapula.

Box 3. Teaching anatomy using visualization.

Adequate skills and knowledge of anatomy are indispensable and should be imparted from the onset of an exercise physiology education. Why not face the reality of mental images in learning anatomy first by closing your eyes and visualizing yourself standing in front of the cadaver. Then, allow your mind's eye to see the anterior deltoid, the pectoralis major, and abdominal muscles. Now, "see" the quadriceps inserting on the tibial tuberosity. Let your mind merge your mental image with physical reality. It is as William Arthur Ward said, *"If you can imagine it, you can achieve it. If you can dream it, you can become it."*

If the furniture in the office or apartment is remembered by having previous knowledge of their position, size, and color, the same "storage" of information is equally true with the study of the body's osteological landmarks. Details about the furniture and the scapula are acquired from images that are subject to scanning in a manner analogous to "seeing" the objects. Each object is scanned, rotated, re-scaled, and mentally transformed and visually manipulated to obtain specific information.

Scanning

Scanning a dissected cadaver is especially critical to accessing information from images. Aside from the visual differences in the radius and the ulna forearm bones, students can also learn to access information in other ways as well. For example, by "scanning" the anterior surface of the radius from the superior aspect to the inferior aspect, students will find that they experience a reduction in time that is consistent with the reality of looking at the actual length of a radius in the lab *versus* the ulna. Scanning not only allows for specific information, such as the radial tuberosity that is located on its proximal, anterior surface, it sets the stage for viewing the image as though the actual length of the forearm and its internal structures exists in the image itself (Box **4**).

Box 4. The significance of cadaver dissection is about the living.

Although cadavers are used in the teaching of gross anatomy, it must be remembered that anatomy is about the living.

There is also a "depth" factor to consider when scanning, for example, the medial and lateral lips of the bicipital groove. With the correct image, students can sense the groove in relation to the elevated positions of the borders. By moving the proximal end of the humerus forward to view the top of the bone, the groove is more pronounced with an obvious demonstration of the 3rd-dimension (depth).

With a second blink, the mind's eye sees the anterior surface of the distal end of the humerus and its relationship with the ulna on the medial and the radius on the lateral side of a supinated forearm and hand. The medial and lateral epicondyles are visualized, which allows for more anatomical views specific to the points of origin for the anterior forearm flexors and the muscles that make up the posterior side of the forearm, respectively.

For example, while scanning from lateral to medial, the muscles in the superficial layer of the forearm can be easily identified. They are the pronator teres, flexor carpi radialis, palmaris longus, and flexor carpi ulnaris. With another blink transformation and scanning of the muscles in the middle layer, the flexor digitorum superficialis muscle is visualized crossing the elbow joint and the wrist to insert on the sides of middle phalanges of digits 2 through 5 (Box **5**).

The mind is the storehouse of anatomical facts and linked information that can be accessed with different images. The key to "seeing" the stored details and particulars begin with the storage process that is primarily in the shape and layout of memorization. For example, regarding the pectoralis major muscle on the right side of the chest, it originates from the proximal anterior two-thirds of the clavicle, the full length of the sternum, and the costal cartilages of ribs one through five. First, the points of origin are visualized. Second, they are stored in memory *via* memorization of the visual location of each anatomical description.

Box 5. Teaching *vs.* research: Which is more important for students?

For several decades, anatomy had a prominent place in physical education, exercise science, and exercise physiology. But, the recent knowledge explosion in the cellular and molecular aspects of human adaptability to sports and regular exercise has had a negative effect on the faculty with an interest in anatomy. The university's emphasis on research *versus* teaching has not helped, and may have been the primary reason for diminishing the interest in the kinesiology (anatomy) courses.

To take the process further, the pectoralis major inserts on the lateral lip of the bicipital groove. Seeing the muscle in this way allows for an understanding of its role in medial rotation of the humerus, given that the muscle shortens (*i.e.,* contracts) toward the points of origin. Note that the origin of the muscle relative to its insertion allows for a mental image of shoulder flexion (with the clavicular fibers) and shoulder extension (with the sternal fibers) among other functions.

Visualizers

Albert Einstein said, "If I can't picture it, I can't understand it." By learning how muscles function from mental pictures, students can be motivated to acquire an interest in anatomy and all types of athletic performances and human movements. "Visualizers" are individuals who have learned to use the power of mental images to recall and remember specific information. They have learned to appreciate the quality of human movement and sports at a level that is rarely matched by athletes who think predominately in words (verbalizers).

Visualizers use mental pictures as a form of seeing and thinking. For example, consider the mental image of a person who is standing in front of you with his back to you. Look through his clothing to see the upper back and, in particular, the left shoulder region. Now, visualize the trapezius, latissimus dorsi, and posterior deltoid muscles in relationship to the dorsal surface of the left scapula. Close your eyes for a moment and then open them, using the blink transformation process to grasp the subtle relationships and interesting bits of anatomical information all healthcare professionals should know and appreciate.

Do you see the left trapezius inserting on the base of the spine of the scapula, throughout the length of the spine of the scapula to the acromion process (a bony process on the scapula)? Note the muscle wasting (*i.e.,* sarcopenia) of the deltoid muscle with its points of the origin from the acromion process (*e.g.,* middle deltoid) and the spine of the scapula (*e.g.,* posterior deltoid) (Box **6**, left side). For comparison, refer to the right side of Box **6** and note the hypertrophy (*i.e.,* muscle enlargement) of the same muscles. Also, note the thickness of the teres major and infraspinatus muscles originate from the dorsal surface of the scapula. Of these two muscles, which one is referred to as the latissimus dorsi's "little helper" in adducting, extending, and inwardly rotating the humerus?

Box 6. The myology of two cadavers.

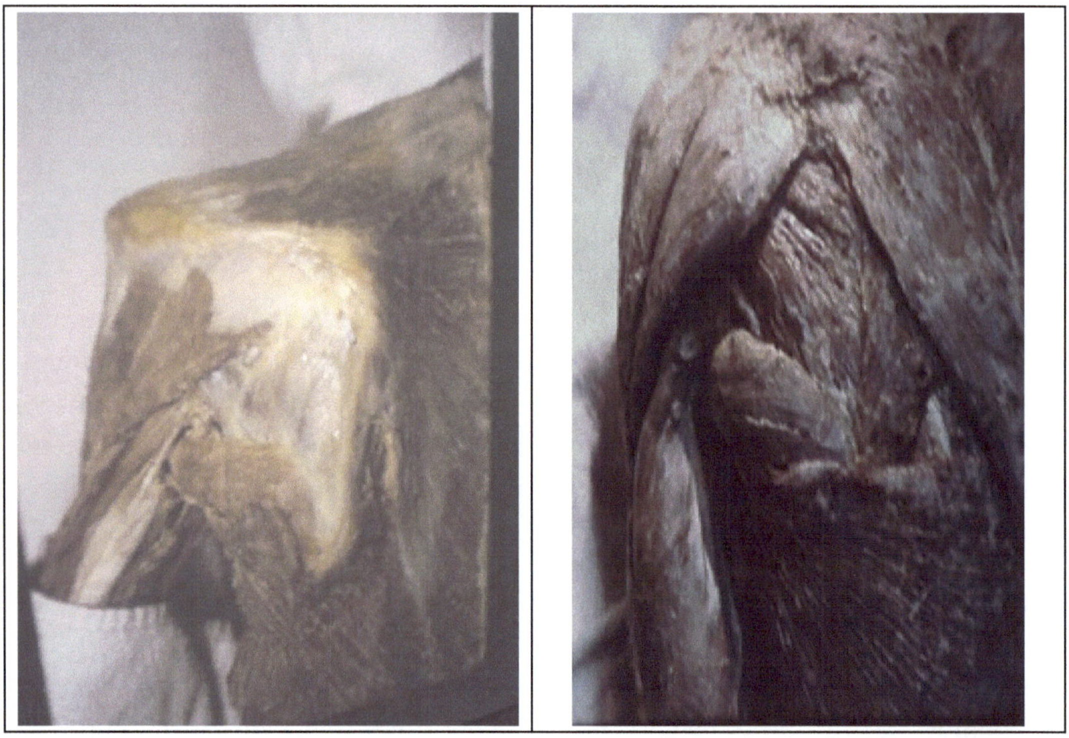

Regarding the anterior view of the left side of the chest, pictured in Box **7**, visualize the origin of the serratus anterior muscle arising from the anterior surface of ribs 1-9. Notice the serrated (*i.e.,* saw-tooth) appearance of the muscle as it originates from the ribs. Now, with a person standing directly in front of you face-to-face, create an image that allows you to visualize the anterior view of the left scapula just behind the thoracic wall. Specifically, look for the anterior surface of the medial border of the left scapula from the superior angle to the inferior angle. This anatomical description is the insertion of the serratus anterior muscle in Box **7**, which is innervated by the long thoracic nerve.

Box 7. The muscles of the left chest, side, and abdomen.

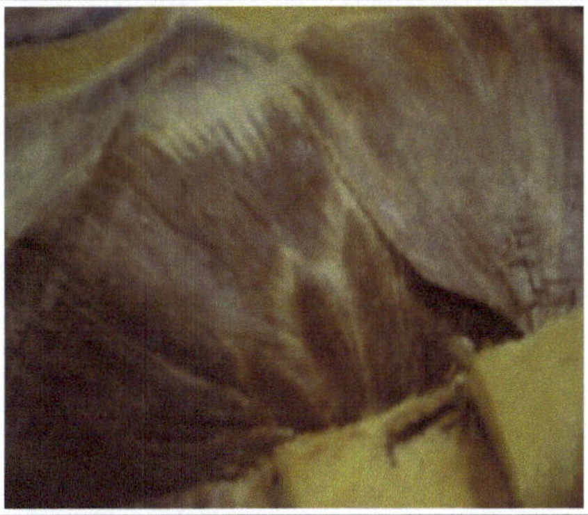

Note the pectoralis major on the left anterior chest wall, which covers the upper origination sites of the serratus anterior. The lower points of origin can be seen arising from the outer surfaces of the rib cage in close articulation with the external oblique muscle as it gives rise to the anterior rectus sheath (in white) that covers the rectus abdominis muscle. If this muscle fails to function, abduction of the upper limb is very difficult. Interestingly, the long thoracic nerve innervates the serratus anterior from a position above the muscle itself, just under the skin and fat layer (in yellow).

Since the muscular system creates forces that exert an action(s) on a less stable bone (*i.e.,* the scapula *vs.* the rib cage), contraction of the serratus anterior results in movement of the scapula towards the left side of the thoracic wall. The movement is referred to as abduction (or protraction), which is a movement of the scapula away from the midline of the body. Hence, the primary purpose of the serratus anterior is to assist the shoulder flexors and abduction by aiding in the upward rotation of the scapula. This comes about by way of two different insertions of the serratus anterior muscle.

The points of origin from ribs 1 through 3 exert an abducting force on the scapula, given that they insert the full length of the medial border of the scapula. The point of origin arising specifically from the outer surfaces of ribs 4 through 9 exert a powerful upward rotation because they insertion primarily on the anterior surface of the inferior angle of the scapula.

The image of the muscle from the anterior point of origin through the chest wall to the scapula allows for a better view of how the muscle assists the anterior deltoid (arising from the anterior distal one-third of the clavicle) and the long head of the biceps brachii (arising from the greater tubercle of the glenoid cavity) to produce full flexion and/or abduction of the upper limb.

Accessing Information

If teachers encourage the use of images in recalling anatomical facts (and even physiological facts), they are encouraging their students to think. When students are asked to think about an image of their car, they can tell you the make, color, and its condition. Information is embedded in the image that may have been forgotten. The image helps in "accessing" (*i.e.,* visualizing the details of what we wish to see. It is the same with seeing the deltoid or the serratus anterior muscles in Box **6** and Box **7**, respectively.

The same can be done with visualizing physiology calculations (Box **8**). As an example, if students are asked in an exercise physiology lab to estimate how much oxygen is necessary to ride a bicycle ergometer at 600 $kpm \cdot min^{-1}$, all that is necessary is to "see" the regression equation: [VO_2 ($L \cdot min^{-1}$) = ($kpm \cdot min^{-1}$ x 2) + 300]. The image provides the answer, which is: 1.5 $L \cdot min^{-1}$. It is the same with determining the subject's cardiac output, using the mental image: [Q ($L \cdot min^{-1}$) = 6.12 x VO_2 ($L \cdot min^{-1}$) + 3.4], which is 12.58 $L \cdot min^{-1}$ (Boone 2014).

Box 8. To visualize is to remember.

Visualizing brings the anatomical bits and physiological pieces to life. It is more than just the use of words. It is engaging one's imagination. When students visualize, they gain insight into the experiences of what they are seeing, feeling, and sensing. Visualization provides a unique perspective that helps in remembering information.

The teacher could instruct the students to create an image of the lungs and their relationship, first, to the atmosphere and, second, the heart. Naturally, it is the teachers' responsibility to present the material in a logical fashion. Then, the students' responsibility is to create the mental images to re-enforce terminology, relationships, and functions. From the air that surrounds the body, an inspired volume of ~500 ml of air fills the lungs with oxygen with each and every breath.

After adjustment for water vapor, picture the respiratory system full of oxygen at a partial pressure of 100 mmHg in contrast to oxygen in the venous blood of 40 mmHg. The resulting pressure gradient is 60 mmHg that produces movement of the oxygen from the respiratory system into the pulmonary capillaries to link with hemoglobin (Hb) to form oxyhemoglobin. At a lung pressure of 100 mmHg and an average of 15 grams of Hb per 100 milliliters (ml) of blood, 20 ml of oxygen is delivered per each 100 ml of blood.

The myocardium pumps the blood saturated with oxygen to the tissues of the muscles. Imagine the flow of the blood from the lungs to the left atrium into the left ventricle. During the contraction of both ventricles with the atrio-ventricular valves shut, the blood is placed under pressure. It is this pressure that propels the blood from the heart into the systemic system.

The vascular structures from the myocardium to the muscles of the left brachium (*i.e.,* arm) include mental images of the aorta connected to the left ventricle, the ascending aorta (which is the extension of the foremost artery from the heart to the arteries of the head, upper body, and the upper limbs), the brachiocephalic trunk, subclavian artery (*i.e.,* the major arteries that furnish the axillary artery in the armpit), and the brachial artery (the chief artery of the arm) that divides into the radial and ulnar arteries of the forearm.

Close your eyes and "see" the arteries just outlined with the smaller arteries arising from each that service related muscles. Visualize the arteries full of oxygen making its way into the smaller arterioles that have adjusted their size by vasodilation to ensure that an ample volume of blood enters the capillaries. The larger lumen size of the arterioles also allows for a reduction in the effort of the left ventricle, thus lowering what is referred to as systemic vascular resistance (or afterload).

With the low resistance to the blood flowing through the arteries and capillaries along with the tissues' need for oxygen, defined by a low partial pressure of 40 mmHg at rest and much lower pressure during exercise, oxygen separates from the Hb molecules and moves from the capillaries into the muscle fibers. Once oxygen is inside the fibers, it is used to develop energy in the form of adenosine triphosphate (ATP) for muscle contraction. Thus, oxygen from the atmosphere (*via* the lungs) becomes the final electron acceptor in the electron transport system of the mitochondria within the muscle fiber.

The point here is that the images allow for the recall of facts that lead to function. The steps involved in muscle contraction can be recalled with a little effort to translate the excitation-coupling process as three or four connected images. The time has come for exercise physiologists to take this information that has revolutionized exercise physiology and merge their thinking with created images. If they are willing to do so, it will transform the way students think, learn, and engage the practice of exercise physiology.

Final Thoughts

The myriad forms of learning with mental images encourages its use, especially in accessing stored information and generating meaning that can be used to take tests, to organize a cardiovascular assessment protocol, or to present a lecture. Mental images, when actively created, are the vital breakthrough point with recalling information at a three-dimensional level as well as the creation of new and meaningful ideas and relationships.

As Thoreau advised, "...if one advances confidently in the direction of his dreams, and endeavors to live the life which he has imagined, he will meet with a success unexpected in common hours." It is logical that the same thinking and outcome is true for success in learning anatomy, exercise physiology, and related key issues.

GLOSSORY

Blink transformations	The decision to let an image disappear while then seeing a new image (*e.g.*, first seeing the image of the long street to your right in front of your house and then, as in a blink of the eye, you see an image of the same street to your left).
Creating images	Using the mind's eye to see an image of what you are thinking about (*e.g.*, think of your apartment or home and you will not only see it, but you can mentally move about the apartment or home from one room to the next while seeing your furniture).
Image rotation	Rotation of an image, such as first seeing in the mind's eye the front of your car and then, by mentally rotating the car, you can see the back of it.
Mental scanning	Occurs when a person, for example, decides to mentally see the driver's side of his or her car and then decides to focus the image specifically first on the front area of the car just above the wheel and then decides to look very closely at first one section and then another section of front left side of the car.

REFERENCES

Boone, T (1990) Imagery and teaching: some reflections. *J Phys Educ, Recreat Dance,* 62, 45-9. [http://dx.doi.org/10.1080/07303084.1990.10604579]

Boone, T (2001) The use of imagery in teaching. *Professionalization of Exercise Physiologyonline.* 4:6, Available from: https://www.asep.org/asep/asep/IMAGERYandEXERCISE PHYSIOLOGY.html

Boone, T (2014) *Introduction to exercise physiology.* Jones & Bartlett Learning, Burlington, Massachusetts.

CHAPTER 7

The Importance of Flexibility Training

Abstract: The quality of professional development of exercise physiologists is determined by the quality of their professional thinking, which in turn is determined by the quality of their critical thinking - for critical thinking is the driving force behind professionalism. Without critical thinking skills, there is little reason to think of exercise physiologists as healthcare professionals. In fact, it is obvious that all the scientific papers, presentations, and posters by exercise physiologists at national and regional meetings cannot define exercise physiology as a profession. This point is within their understanding if they work at critical thinking as they have taught their students to think scientifically. Yet, many exercise physiologists continue to present their scientific papers without internalizing the concepts and principles essential to the underlying concepts of critical thinking and professionalism in exercise physiology. Despite having the doctorate degree and after teaching years of college and university courses, it is apparent that relatively few professors have the desire to become self-directed, self-monitored, and self-corrective critical thinkers to guide their students' path towards a professional understanding of flexibility training.

Keywords: Adaptive shortening, Adductors, Flexibility training, Hamstrings, Myocardial oxygen consumption, Oxygen transport, Plantar flexors, Stretching exercises.

INTRODUCTION

During my first year of college, I decided that I wanted to be a gymnast. What I did not know was the importance of flexibility in learning gymnastics. I thought that gymnastics was all about strength and determination. I learned rather quickly that while both are important, being a gymnast meant that I needed above average flexibility. I had become rather strong from years of football training and lifting weights. Baseball and various track and field events (such as pole vaulting and

Tommy Boone

low hurdles) helped me develop the ability to focus my attention and perform with a certain degree of skill. But, in terms of the required range of motion a gymnast should have, I was at rock bottom. Forget about dropping into a side splits or even touching my toes from a standing position, I simply did not have the flexibility to do so.

The idea of training for flexibility in the same way one trains for strength or to run faster was not part of my earlier athletics and yet, it is clear in retrospect that if I had been more flexible I would have achieved more in gymnastics (Boone 1971). For certain, I would have been able to avoid certain injuries that delayed maximizing my gymnastic abilities. Also, with increased flexibility, I would have been physically prepared to be a better all-around gymnast (Box **1**).

Box 1. Flexibility training.

Flexibility is defined as the allowed range of motion at any given joint throughout the skeletal and muscular structures. There cannot be any question that everyone, especially athletes must engage in flexibility training.

As you might understand, my first year as a gymnast at Northwestern State University in Natchitoches, LA was a difficult period of mental and physical adjustment. I was strong so strength skills were easy to perform. Also, I was determined and eventually I learned to perform at a certain level. I learned the gymnastics skills very quickly, which helped me to stay motivated. However, it did not take too long to figure out that without the flexibility to perform certain gymnastic moves, being successful as an all-around gymnast was not possible.

When a gymnast fails to have the range of movement in a joint or series of joints to do, for example, a side splits, the athletic performance is constrained by the limitation in joint motion. In short, this means that either the performance is not possible or it is performed below an acceptable standard. To perform the skill with the desired execution, the athlete's degree of suppleness of the muscles and related connective tissues must be increased. Therefore, the objective is to engage the athlete in flexibility training with the same vigor as one would do for strength, speed, and endurance training.

Knowledge of not only the specifics of the sport is important, but also an understanding of the body and how it moves. As an example, when performing on the parallel bars, it is standard practice to perform an "L" support (*i.e.,* while in the upright position on the bars, the lower limbs are raised to the horizontal position). If the gymnast has difficulty in raising the lower limbs (legs) to the "L" position, is the problem too little strength in the hip flexors or too little flexibility in the hamstrings? Or, is the problem specific to the strength of the quadriceps? Perhaps, it is the gymnast's inability to perform dynamically (also called dynamic or kinetic flexibility)? Is it a problem of static-active flexibility (*i.e.,* the agonists lift the lower limbs while the antagonists are being stretched)?

Understanding the way in which muscles originate and insert on specific bones, and how they function individually and collectively help the athlete figure out the right answer to the question is part of coaching athletes. For example, if the hip flexors are weak, what is the best way to strengthen them? If it is poor flexibility of the hamstring muscles, how long will it take to increase the range of motion at the hips (Box **2**)? What is the best stretching exercise to increase the range of motion of the muscles that arise from the ischial tuberosity? Without the right information, the gymnast may try to strengthen the hip flexors to compensate for the poor hip flexion and, therefore, fail to correct the lack of range of motion in the posterior thigh muscles (*i.e.,* the hamstring muscles in particular).

Box 2. Factors that distract from flexibility.

Aside from failing to systematic trained to develop a greater range of motion, there are certain factors that distract from flexibility. They are the different joint structures, the size of the individual muscles, and the related connective tissue. There is also the question of motivation to do what is necessary to be more flexible. It is important that static stretching be performed more so than dynamic stretching, especially during the warm-up.

While coaches and athletes understand the importance of muscle strength, speed, and endurance, developing flexibility is often reduced to whatever time is left in the exercise program (*e.g.,* the last 5 minutes of a 60-minute workout is dedicated to flexibility training). Given that flexibility training is important, one would assume that coaches, athletes, and exercise physiologists are aware of the best means to increasing the athletes' range of motion?

But, unfortunately, they are either not interested in flexibility training or do not understand it. The result is a decrease in movement efficiency and the ability of athletes to learn specific skills. And yet, just 30 minutes of static stretching three times a week will significantly improve flexibility, lower the chance of muscle, tendon, and/or joint injuries, and optimize the efficiency of the athlete's performance (Boone 1976). In short, an adequate range of motion is critical to the success of the athlete.

The Benefits

While it is common practice to focus on the physiology of athletics, it is less common that athletes train for flexibility. The emphasis in this book is on flexibility training (*i.e.,* the anatomy of the body), particularly static stretching. The purpose is to present the anatomical concepts necessary in understanding the muscles that need stretching and why. One benefit of an adequate range of motion whether throwing a baseball, doing a back flip on a trampoline, or sprinting in a race is that the execution will be less awkward and exhaustive (Fletcher & Jones 2004; Sayers *et al.* 2008). With the right range of motion in the muscles and joints, there will be less soreness and injury, and the increased likelihood of a successful performance (Young *et al.* 2004; Witvrouw *et al.* 2003).

Without flexibility the simplest of athletic endeavors (such as jogging) cannot be performed with efficiency (Box **3**). Professional athletes and individuals with restricted joint motion understand that flexibility is important. They realize that if you do not have the range of motion required to perform an athletic skill, then the performance will suffer. Take, for example, in the latter case, a person with severely limited range of motion due to a specific joint disease or connective tissue that restricts flexibility. This person expends a lot of wasted energy when jogging. The muscles are unable to relax and allow for the natural unfolding of the sequential aspects of jogging. Also, there is the likelihood of too much stress on certain muscles while other muscles act to restrict motion (such as the hip flexors that do not allow for adequate hip extension) (Godges *et al.* 1989).

Box 3. Lack of training is unsafe.

It is natural that the muscles of athletes lose strength, size and flexibility when not in training. As a result, athletes are more prone to joint and muscle injuries when they don't take the time to train properly for a greater range of motion. Adaptive shortening is the gradual to acute loss of the muscles' ability to relax and accommodate the intended range of motion across a joint.

A byproduct of this type of restricted flexibility is an increased load placed on the cardiovascular system. Heart rate (HR) and systolic blood pressure (SBP) are likely to be increased, which will increase the work of the heart. This is easily illustrated by calculating myocardial oxygen consumption (MVO_2), using the following formula: MVO_2 = .14 (HR x SBP x .01) – 6.3

$$\begin{aligned} MVO_2 &= .14\ (HR \times SBP \times .01) - 6.3 \\ &= .14\ (130 \times 160 \times .01) - 6.3 \\ &= 22.82\ mL \cdot 100\ g\ LV \cdot min^{-1}\ \text{(with flexibility training)} \end{aligned}$$

$$\begin{aligned} MVO_2 &= .14\ (HR \times SBP \times .01) - 6.3 \\ &= .14\ (160 \times 190 \times .01) - 6.3 \\ &= 36.26\ mL \cdot 100\ g\ LV \cdot min^{-1}\ \text{(without flexibility training)} \end{aligned}$$

Note that without flexibility, the work of the jogger's heart is increased due to the difficulty of overcoming the inertia of the muscles that lack the range of motion to accommodate the jogging exercise. Unfortunately, the possibility exists that among middle-aged jogger's with heart disease, the increased effort increases HR and SBP that, then, increases to a critical point requiring more oxygen than the coronary arteries can supply the heart. Even if the arteries are moderately obstructed under conditions of increased need for oxygen, it is very likely that a negative result will occur (*e.g.,* angina pectoris, *i.e.,* chest pain due to ischemia) in association with the loss of body efficiency (Boone 2014).

Flexibility is Important

Being flexible reduces the possibility of an injury, both musculoskeletal and cardiovascular. It sets the stage for improving athletic performance. The athlete's muscles perform more with less tension, thus allowing for increased coordination and agility. As a result, exercises such as jogging, running, dancing, throwing, or kicking can be performed with finesse when the range of movement in a joint or a series of joints is attainable without an increased effort.

Although flexibility is specific to each joint, it is likely that this point has been over-emphasized with regard to joints that seldom ever experience increased tightness. For example, there is little reason to spend time stretching the wrist flexors and/or extensors. The muscles that arise predominately from the medial epicondyle (forearm flexors) and lateral epicondyle (forearm extensors) do not undergo adaptive shortening. Yet, it is common knowledge that the primary hip flexor muscles (psoas major and iliacus), thigh adductor muscles (pectineus, adductor longus, adductor brevis, and gracilis), and lower back muscles (erector spinae) do undergo adaptive shortening (Box **4**). Therefore, it is logical that these muscles need stretching (Boone 2014).

Box 4. Lack of exercise leads to loss of flexibility.

When muscles and connective tissues attaching to bones are not stretched to their normal limits, they become less stretchable resulting in a decrease in flexibility.

When muscles are allowed to shorten (without contraction), the muscles adapt to the decrease in their range of motion. “Adaptive shortening” is the term used to explain the gradual to acute loss of the muscles' ability to accommodate the desired range of motion across a joint. The decrease is typically characterized as an increased tenseness in the connective tissue that is part of the structure of muscles. There may also be an increase in muscle tone that hinders relaxation of the muscle under conditions of increased need for a greater range of motion. The end result is an increase in the likelihood of tearing a muscle that is resisting the need to stretch. Several prominent muscles that undergo adaptive shortening are:

- The pectoralis major, coracobrachialis, and the short head of the biceps brachii muscles of the anterior chest wall and shoulder joint due to the tendency to slump the shoulders forward when positioning the upper limbs in front of the body (as in typing at work on a computer).
- The psoas major and the iliacus muscles of the transverse processes of the lumbar vertebrae and the anterior surface of the ilium, respectively, due to the habitual sitting and anterior convexity of the lower spine.

- The five adductors (pectenius, adductor longus, gracilis, adductor brevis, and anterior fibers of the adductor magnus) located on the inside of the thigh due to the relatively little need to abduct the lower extremities when sitting or standing.
- The three hamstring muscles (semitendinous, semimembranous, and the long head of the biceps femoris) resist being stretched due to the habitual act of sitting with the knees flexed, and
- The gastrocnemius and soleus complex (calf muscles) given that these muscles are often over used in the plantar flexed position of women who wear high-heeled footwear.

After years of sedentary living coupled with the typical daily lifestyle postures, these muscles and related fascia undergo adaptive shortening. The endomysium (fascia sheath that envelops individual fibers), perimysium (fascia that binds groups of muscle fibers into individual fasciculi), and epimysium (fascia sheath that binds entire fascicles) become progressively tighter and shorten with a decrease in range of motion. Thus, when bending forward (*i.e.,* flexing at the hips), as when touching one's toes or picking up the morning paper, the poor range of motion of the hamstrings resist the natural tendency of the pelvic region to rotate forward and downward. The resistance in the muscles indicates that the expected (or maximal) range of motion is decreased.

While not all flexibility problems can be traced to this one example, it is the primary way in which flexibility is lost. Its simplicity also suggests the means to which the problem of less joint mobility (or flexibility) can be corrected. That is, if a particular posture is determined to have created certain negative conditions about a joint or joints, correcting the posture should correct the problem. Hence, all the hypothetical person has to do is to stop sitting so much. However, that may not be possible since most employees must perform much of what they do while sitting on a daily basis. What is possible is this: First, the decision to slow the adaptation by occasionally standing up and engaging in flexibility exercises that address the involved muscles. Second, the decision to engage in a full range of motion exercises after work to increase and maintain flexibility (Box **5**).

Unfortunately, it is common knowledge that neither recommendation is followed. As an example, many people today still complain of backaches. The pain is due to the tightness of the low back and hamstring muscles that limit range of motion when bending forward at the hips. It is strange why instructors of aerobic dance, personal trainers at health and wellness centers, and rehabilitation specialists for the middle-aged and elderly fail to understand this point.

Box 5. The objective of flexibility training.

The objective of flexibility training is to produce changes in muscle's fascia sheaths. There is little need to address limitations imposed by the design of the skeletal system or the properties that constitute the joint capsule, ligaments, and tendons.

With just a few minutes of stretching every day, joint pain often ceases to exist as normal motion is restored. This restoration means that the stiffness of the related connective tissues and the tendency for the muscles to resist stretch when not relaxed have undergone positive adaptations to accommodate a greater motion in the low back and hamstring complex. There is still the question of identifying exercises to improve muscle power and muscle endurance. But, at least the muscles are at an acceptable level of flexibility, and they can now function with less stress on the cardiovascular system.

A well-designed flexibility routine is directed at positive changes in the muscles about the joints and the connective tissues that hold the muscles fibers together, but not so much with the ligaments, tendons, and joint capsule. These latter structures are essentially non-elastic while muscle tissue has the capacity to stretch more than twice its length without sustaining critical damage. Tendons have tremendous tensile strength and, therefore, are virtually inelastic.

It may also be necessary to direct one's attention to signals that suggest a reduction in the extensibility of muscle as a function of emotions and stress. For example, when the muscles at the neck are tight (such as the trapezius, in particular), there is very likely the need to correct or minimize the impact of the mental and/or emotional stressors. This is especially true for athletic conditions in which the athlete's performance suffers from apprehension and stress.

While the development of flexibility is a slow process, the benefits are worth the commitment. In fact, without the desire to be more flexible and the willingness to stay with a flexibility routine, most gymnastic skills would simply be impossible to execute. On the other hand, with adequate range of motion, gymnasts are able to reach further, bend deeper, and move with less energy expended throughout a full range of motion. Flexibility training is especially important during periods of inactivity (Box **6**). When done correctly, it allows for a meaningful experience in athletics, whether gymnastics, track and field, handball, tennis, or soccer.

Box 6. Training for increased flexibility.

One of the reasons that muscles lose their flexibility is from inactivity. If it continues for a long time, the loss of flexibility could lead to a permanent loss of certain movements and clinically important changes in posture and normal muscle function. Static active flexibility is the ability to stretch an antagonist muscle using only the tension in the agonist muscle. Now, having said that, think about this. The average person does not think of flexibility as an important part of overall fitness. Part of the reason why lies with the lack of an education about fitness, particularly flexibility training. To develop a greater range of motion, static stretches should be held for 30 seconds, possibly up to 60 seconds, to gain a benefit, and the stretches should be performed regularly, ideally twice a day, every day or at minimal once a day, every other day.

The impact of flexibility training goes beyond athletics. It improves breathing by increasing the capacity of the chest to enlarge, which has a direct effect on the function of the lungs. They are able to bring in a larger volume of air per breath. This volume is called the tidal volume (T_V), which at rest is usually about 500 ml of air with each breath. What is seldom realized is that the size of the T_V is more important than the frequency of breaths (F_b) per minute.

Breathing (*i.e.*, expired ventilation, V_E) is more efficient with an increase in T_V and a decrease F_b. Physiologically, this relationship between the two variables helps to explain the importance of T_V to alveolar ventilation (V_A). The latter [V_A = (T_V – anatomic dead space of 150 mL) x F_b] is how much fresh air enters the distal parts of the lungs, the alveoli, which is at rest (500 – 150) = 350 x 12 or 4.2 $L \cdot min^{-1}$ of the resting 6 $L \cdot min^{-1}$ V_E].

The V_A of 4.2 $L \cdot min^{-1}$ diffuses across the alveoli-capillary membrane to associate with hemoglobin. Hence, the transport of oxygen in the blood (oxyhemoglobin, HbO_2) to all the tissues of the body is dependent in part on the range of motion of the thorax and chest muscles. Why, because a decrease in thoracic and/or chest muscle range of motion decreases T_V that requires F_b to increase to sustain V_E? The end result is a decrease in V_A (Boone 2014).

Oxygen transport in the blood is also affected by the condition of skeletal muscles, especially whether they are relaxed (elastic) or stiff (inelastic). The blood flows more easily through relaxed muscles than tense muscles. The lack of tension allows for an increase in blood flow and, therefore, an increase in oxygen and energy (adenosine triphosphate, ATP) at the cellular level for sustaining if not increasing muscle contraction. There is also a decrease in the tendency of the byproduct of glucose (lactic acid) to remain in the active muscles. Both metabolic conditions help to maximize the function of muscles and the overall physical performance of the recreational subject or athlete.

Flexibility training has a positive influence on energy production and cellular function. This is realized by improving chemical energy and by changing the internal environment of the cell from more acid to less acid. Without question, suppleness and resilience are important features of muscle fibers when it comes to the production force needed to run, dance, and swim with ease and efficiency. Perhaps, the most obvious conclusion is that the increase in flexibility provides a significant decrease in resistance to moving. With appropriate training (defined as "good" flexibility exercises), anyone can develop an increase in flexibility. It is not just a factor of disuse, overuse, age, or any number of other potentially confounding factors. There is also the factor of a "good" flexibility exercise and a "useless" flexibility exercise.

The Concerns

If flexibility training is good, what are the concerns? The concerns stem from the fact that it is commonplace for athletes and others to use the wrong techniques in effort to develop flexibility. They are also taught many exercises that are useless and/or dangerous. Why this point remains such a common problem is consistent with the fact that the majority of the coaches, trainers, and exercise physiologists are not well educated in anatomy. They lead, teach, and/or engage in flexibility exercises in accordance with traditional practices. As a result, they do not know which exercises to use, how long they should be used, or why. As an example, consider the following questions about aerobic dance:

- Which flexibility exercises should be included in the warm-up session prior to dancing?
- Which exercises should be excluded from the dance session?
- How should certain exercises be performed?
- Which exercises should be performed after dancing?
- How much time should be given to each exercise before and after dancing?

These questions apply to all sports, including gymnastics, football, and basketball. They also apply to the middle-aged jogger. Being able to answer these questions adds credibility to the athletic and/or fitness programs. Too often though there are few if any qualified individuals to help athletes and/or others interested in an effective and safe stretching routine. All athletes, beginners through elite levels, need sound advice and guidance is the use of stretching exercises just as they need credible information regarding muscle strength development and cardiovascular training (Box 7).

Box 7. Not all athletes are the same.

Stretching is the key to increasing the range of motion in muscles. But, please appreciate that some athletes are more flexible than other athletes. Even so, it is possible for all athletes to increase their flexibility with the right training, and this is especially true if they are dedicated to a regular regimen of stretching.

Maximizing athletic potential is simply not possible with poor or unsafe teaching or coaching techniques. This is true when athletes and/or participants are placed in positions to achieve limb and body postures beyond usual limits of motion. Understanding this point and taking the necessary steps to hire qualified coaches, instructors, and exercise physiologists are essential to a safe stretching program.

When using a safe, "good", and effective stretching routine, it can help with the following considerations:

- It can help correct the negative effects of poor posture.
- It can improve performance, athletic or otherwise.
- It can aid in the development of other physical fitness factors.
- It can improve the function of the musculoskeletal system.

- It can decrease the likelihood of low back pain.
- It can improve the efficiency of the physiological function of the body.
- It can help with the muscle soreness that often results from athletics and/or various work conditions.
- It can increase an ease of movement whether it is sports or life in general.
- It can increase reaction time.
- It can reduce the risk of injury.
- It can increase the feeling of control over body movements.
- It can improve posture and efficiency of movement.
- It can delay the onset of muscular fatigue.
- It can increase the athlete's skill level and muscular efficiency.

Final Thoughts

The focus on physiology in athletics is so common a topic of research that it has diminished the study of anatomy and flexibility. And yet, without the range of motion throughout the musculoskeletal system to move efficiently, there is an increase in the work of the cardiovascular system. This increase in work is a function of the necessity to overcome the inertia of the muscles to accommodate human movement. Conversely, being flexible helps to reduce the possibility of various musculoskeletal and/or cardiovascular injuries. Also, it sets the stage for improving athletic performance and life in general, given that the muscles perform more efficiently with increased coordination and agility.

While the development of flexibility is a slow process, the benefits are well worth the commitment of 15 to 20 minutes of static stretching at least three times a week. But, there are several concerns. For example, it is common for athletes and others to use the wrong techniques in their desire to develop a greater range of motion. Unfortunately, they are also taught exercises that are useless and/or dangerous. Why this point remains such a common problem is consistent with the fact that the majority of the coaches, fitness instructors, trainers, and exercise physiologists are not well educated in anatomy.

GLOSSORY

Adaptive shortening	Muscle tightness that occurs due to muscles remaining in a shortened position for a long period of time.

Adductors	A muscle whose contraction results in the movement of a limb or other part of the body toward the midline of the body or toward another part of the body.
Flexibility training	Execution of stretching exercises for the purpose of increasing one's range of motion.
Hamstrings	Muscles on the posterior side of the thigh.
Oxygen transport	Process by which oxygen carried by red blood cell to the peripheral tissues.
Plantar flexors	Muscles that originate predominately on the posterior aspect of the leg that produce with contraction a downward pointing of the foot and toes.
Stretching exercises	Form of exercise in which muscles are placed on stretch to improve the muscles' range of motion.

REFERENCES

Boone, T (1971) Hints for better gymnastic performance. *Coaching Clinic,* 9, 15-6.

Boone, T (1976) *Illustrated handbook of gymnastics, tumbling, and trampolining.* Parker Publishing Company, West Nyack, New York.

Boone, T (2014) *Introduction to exercise physiology.* Jones & Bartlett Learning, Burlington, Massachusetts.

Fletcher, IM & Jones, B (2004) The effect of different warm-up stretch protocols on 20 meter sprint performance in trained rugby union players. *J Strength Cond Res,* 18, 885-8.
[PMID: 15574098]

Godges, JJ, Macrae, H, Longdon, C, Tinberg, C & Macrae, PG (1989) The effects of two stretching procedures on hip range of motion and gait economy. *J Orthop Sports Phys Ther,* 10, 350-7.
[http://dx.doi.org/10.2519/jospt.1989.10.9.350] [PMID: 18791317]

Sayers, AL, Farley, RS, Fuller, DK, Jubenville, CB & Caputo, JL (2008) The effect of static stretching on phases of sprint performance in elite soccer players. *J Strength Cond Res,* 22, 1416-21.
[http://dx.doi.org/10.1519/JSC.0b013e318181a450] [PMID: 18714249]

Witvrouw, E, Danneels, L, Asselman, P, DHave, T & Cambier, D (2003) Muscle flexibility as a risk factor for developing muscle injuries in male professional soccer players. A prospective study. *Am J Sports Med,* 31, 41-6.
[PMID: 12531755]

Young, W, Clothier, P, Otago, L, Bruce, L & Liddell, D (2004) Acute effects of static stretching on hip flexor and quadriceps flexibility, range of motion and foot speed in kicking a football. *J Sci Med Sport,* 7, 23-31.
[http://dx.doi.org/10.1016/S1440-2440(04)80040-9] [PMID: 15139161]

CHAPTER 8

Methods of Flexibility Training

Abstract: Flexibility refers to the range of motion of the musculoskeletal system. It is trainable, but only when it is done correctly. Warming-up should not be confused with training for an increase in range of motion. Flexibility is a logical prerequisite to performing athletic skills with ease, efficiency, and safety. If stretching is done on a regular basis, there will be an increase in the range of motion at specific joints. The stretching will help to improve human movement, whether it is athletics or engaging in physical activity, the circulation of blood and oxygen to the active tissues, and the pain and soreness that results from using the muscles. In general, there are four methods to increase and maintain flexibility: (1) static stretching; (2) ballistic (or dynamic) stretching; (3) contract-relax stretching (also called PNF, proprioceptive neuromuscular facilitation); and (4) passive stretching.

Keywords: Ballistic stretching, Contract-relax stretching, Human movement, Muscle soreness, Passive stretching, Static stretching.

INTRODUCTION

There are three popular methods to increase and/or maintain flexibility: (1) static stretching; (2) ballistic (or dynamic) stretching; and (3) contract-relax stretching (also called PNF, proprioceptive neuromuscular facilitation). These stretching methods can be done alone without additional help from a partner or special exercise device. A fourth method is referred to as passive stretching. It involves the use of external force that is usually provided by a partner to apply the additional pressure to achieve and/or maintain a range of motion throughout the musculoskeletal system.

Static Stretching

Static stretching is the slow and continuous holding of a stretched position. It is

Tommy Boone

the most common method of stretching. It is the method most commonly used by gymnasts and dancers. Most users believe it is as effective as the other methods for increasing flexibility. There are several advantages of static stretching when compared to ballistic stretching, which involves bobbing, bouncing, and rhythmic types of movements to position muscles and joints through a progressively greater range of motion (Box **1**) (Boone 2014).

Box 1. Static stretching.

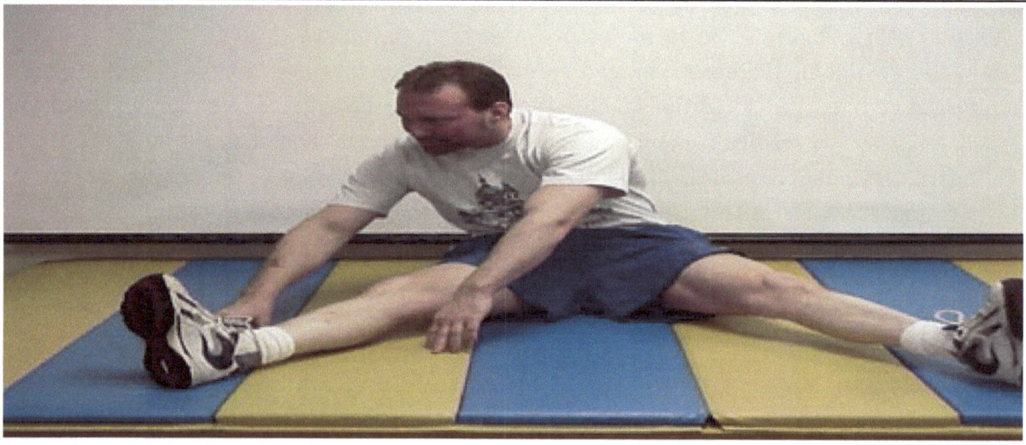

The static stretch is also referred to as the static-passive stretch whereby a person assumes a position and holds it with some part of the body or with the assistance of a partner. It remains an effective, relatively safe, and popular method of stretching. The static method allows for the elastic components of the connective tissues to lengthen very slowly with little danger of damage. This method is also known as the slow stretch and hold method in which, following the stretch, the position is held for 10 to 30 seconds (or even longer, such as 60 seconds). Stretching of the muscles as far as they will go and holding the position stimulates the muscles and related structures to relax and elongate.

When the stretching of a muscle group is at its farthest point, the position is maintained. It should be done slowly and carefully. When done correctly, there is very little likelihood of injury to the muscles and/or connective tissues. The stretching exercises are usually performed without the help of another person or device, which decreases the danger of going beyond the safe range of motion. The exercises are simple, easy to perform, and result in the less energy expended, which leaves energy to perform other activities. When the stretch is held long enough at its farthest point, it can induce muscle relaxation *via* the firing of the Golgi tendon organs (GTOs). These are important advantages and differences between the slow, controlled stretch of the relaxed muscles and the bouncing type (ballistic) stretching exercises.

A slight variation of the static stretch method is used by experienced athletes who perform an additional stretch that goes beyond the initial stretch-hold position. In this case, the static stretch is comprised of two parts. Firstly, the initial stretching and holding position, which takes 10 to 30 seconds or longer. Secondly, then stretch slightly further and hold for another 10 to 30 seconds or longer. The second part is often referred to as the developmental stretch. If the first part is done correctly, then, it is not necessary to over-stretch. In fact, this second part could set the stage for an injury and should not be done until the temperature of muscles and the lubrication around the joints are increased. This is why it is best done during the cool-down phase while the body temperature is still elevated.

Ballistic Stretching

Ballistic stretching (also referred to as dynamic stretching) consists of using the momentum of the body or a limb in bouncing, bobbing, swinging, rebounding, or rapid warm-up calisthenics movements to increase flexibility, whether controlled or uncontrolled (Box **2**). There are many examples of this type of stretching in fitness centers and throughout the sports programs. One popular ballistic stretch is the person who stands with the knees straight, leans forward, and bounces several times in effort to reach further each time to touch the toes.

Box 2. Ballistic stretching.

Ballistic stretching is generally not considered as wise or useful in creating a greater range of motion. Failing to allow the muscles and associated tissues adjust to the bouncing, there is an increased likelihood of injury.

Interestingly enough, most athletes are not aware of the fact that ballistic stretching increases the chances of an injury. Actually, it does not take very many red flags to realize that the bouncing down repeatedly toward the toes, for example, results in excessive loading of the muscles across the posterior aspect of hips and knees. There is no secret that ballistic stretching may cause damage to the connective tissues when forced to stretch beyond their elastic capabilities.

The problem with ballistic stretching is that the extensibility of a group of muscles is a large unknown factor that varies according to certain conditions. At times, it seems that no matter how much jerking or pulling going on, the muscles adjust and there are no injuries. But, as life goes and when least expected, a small almost insignificant jerk or bounce can result in muscle soreness and injury. This unknown factor alone is an important reason to avoid the ballistic stretch method.

Another reason has to do with the tendency for the muscles to protect themselves by contracting when bouncing. The increased tension in response to the stretch-reflex creates a greater resistance to the stretching of the muscles. The result is a greater expenditure of energy with each exercise, and a greater risk of damage. Regardless of these disadvantages, there are several reasons why athletes use the ballistic stretching technique (Boone 2014):

- First, the ballistic stretch method does in fact increase musculoskeletal range of motion (*i.e.*, flexibility).
- Second, given the ballistic nature of most athletic skills and the acquisition of specific components, it may be the right method for increasing flexibility during the dynamics of learning certain sport skills. This point should be taken into consideration when the ballistic approach to stretching is modified to avoid bouncing or jerky movements.

PNF Stretching

There are two major types of proprioceptive neuromuscular facilitation stretching or PNF stretching. First, there is the contract-relax (hold-relax) method and, second, the contract-relax-contract (hold-relax-contract) method. Both methods are primarily therapeutic techniques to improve range of motion. The idea is that a muscle is better able to relax after a contraction.

Take the hamstring muscles for example. The posterior thigh muscles are placed on a slight stretch for 5 seconds followed by an isometric contraction for 5 seconds. Then, the muscle group is relaxed followed by a second static stretch in which the muscle group is stretched even further while relaxed.

This method has been shown to increase flexibility by working with rather than against the stretch reflex syndrome. The contraction of the muscle group before it is stretched signals the muscles to relax by way of the inverse stretch reflex that is located in the tendons. The reduction in resistance results in an improvement in range of motion during the lengthening stretch (Boone 2014).

The PNF exercises are done alone or with a partner to provide resistance against the isometric phase, and later to passively take the joint through an increased range of motion. The following steps characterize the stretching method:

1. Lie flat on the back with the right lower limb straight up in the air. The objective is to increase the range of motion of the muscles on the posterior aspect of the right thigh (*i.e.,* the hamstrings) to allow the lower limb to move closer to the chest.
2. With the right lower limb is raised (*i.e.,* flexed at the hip), the position of the limb (or point of tightness) is determined primarily by the resistance realized in the hip extensors (*e.g.,* semitendinosus, semimembranosus, long head of the biceps femoris, and the vertical fibers of the adductor magnus).
3. Pulling the lower limb closer to the chest results in the subjective feeling of pain. However, it is possible to realize a greater range of motion of the resisting muscles (hamstrings) by doing the contract-relax method.
4. Reach up and grasp the right leg about the calf region with both hands. While holding the leg, try to move the lower limb back towards the floor or mat.
5. The hamstring muscles contract, but the leg remains motionless while experiencing an isometric contraction. After 5 to 10 seconds of stretching, relax the hamstrings and move the leg again toward the chest. Note that the second attempt to place the lower limb close to the chest is usually realized with a greater range of motion.

The PNF exercises are thought to be an excellent method to increase flexibility. But, the literature is mixed when it comes to the notion that the method helps to reset the stretch reflex level with a resulting increase in muscle relaxation. What is generally agreed upon, however, is that the method is associated with increased risk of injury. Also, when compared to the static stretch method, the contract-relax method has several additional drawbacks. One in particular is when using partner-assisted stretching (Box **3**), communication between the person being stretched and the person applying external force on the muscles is essential.

Box 3. Stretch without pain.

Stretching should not result in pain. When done correctly, it can prevent injury by relaxing the muscles as they go through a greater range of motion.

Passive Stretching

Passive stretching requires two conditions. Firstly, the client and/or athlete is placed in a relaxed position, thus it is often referred to as "relaxed stretching". Secondly, an external force is applied by another person (*e.g.,* coach, athletic trainer, or exercise physiologist) or by an apparatus. When done correctly, it is very effective in improving flexibility and relieving spasms in muscles after an injury. Stretches should be done regularly (*e.g.,* twice a day, every day). Under no circumstances should the stretches be painful. Instead, the subject should feel a mild-intensity during the stretch and, then, maintain the position for 20 to 60 seconds. When the tension eases up, the stretch can be taken little further. Repeating this process increases flexibility, but when done improperly, as when too much force is applied, the stretching may increase the likelihood of muscle soreness and injury (Boone 2014).

Final Thoughts

Without question, flexibility training is the least understood of all the fitness components. That is why there is much confusion about which method should be used for athletes of different sports and for non-athletes. Both the static and the ballistic methods result in a greater range of motion. The static method is likely to bring about a decrease in the passive tension of the muscle more so than the ballistic method. As the muscle relaxes and allows for a greater range of movement, less external force has to be applied.

In addition to the method used to obtain a greater range of motion, there are various factors that influence stretching. For example, not all joints in the body are equally susceptible to flexibility training. There is a certain amount of internal resistance within a joint and the bony structures that limit movement. The athlete also has to be mindful of the temperature of the joints and the associated tissues, the elasticity of muscle tissue, tendons, and ligaments, and the temperature where the stretching routine is taking place. As to the latter factor, it is clear that warmer temperatures result in a greater range of motion than colder temperatures. Then, too, it is important to remember that athletes are generally more flexible in the afternoon than in the morning, pre-adolescents are more flexible than adults, and females are more flexible than males.

GLOSSORY

Ballistic stretch	A form of dynamic stretching using a bouncing motion that if not done correctly can cause injury.
Golgi tendon organ	A nerve receptor found in tendons.
Passive stretch	A form of static stretching during which an external force is applied on a limb to move it into the new position.
Static stretch	Stretching of a muscle group that is challenging but comfortable for somewhere between 10 to 30 seconds.

REFERENCES

Boone, T (2014) *Introduction to exercise physiology*. Jones & Bartlett Learning, Burlington, Massachusetts.

CHAPTER 9

Developing a Flexibility Program

Abstract: Improving flexibility is primarily the result of performing stretching exercises. The right flexibility program will provide the athlete with the knowledge to increase range of motion, maximize efficiency of movement, supplement training, and enhance recovery. A good flexibility program concentrates on muscle groups most likely to experience adaptive shortening. In the majority of the cases, just three flexibility exercises will produce the range of motion required to optimize the musculoskeletal system for almost any sport. Be sure to remember that there are "good, useless, and dangerous" flexibility exercises. The useless and the dangerous exercises must be avoided. An excellent example of the latter point is the hurdler's stretch exercise during which the position of the knee and leg stretches the medial collateral ligament while putting pressure on the medial meniscus.

Keywords: Anatomy, Flexibility training, Hamstring muscles, Musculoskeletal joint, Muscle spindles.

INTRODUCTION

It is assumed that the athlete, coach, and/or exercise physiologist understands the ethical and practical reasons for flexibility training. Let us also assume that the static method of flexibility training is chosen as the method to increase flexibility. Implied in the decision is that the stretching exercises are important to maximize performance, and that static stretching is the preferred training method since it is safe. The protection of clients and patients must be held as the highest priority.

Since academic exercise physiologists cannot afford to produce negligent graduates, it is not necessary to push the musculoskeletal joint to the point of pain during stretching. Feeling the tension of the stretch is good, but not pain. Staying injury-free with predictable benefits require a proper stretching program. Aside

Tommy Boone

from the mental benefit of being prepared, the musculoskeletal benefits are increased range of motion, decreased muscle stress, decreased muscle soreness, decreased risk of injury, improved circulation, improved sports performance, and good posture.

To get these benefits, the following assumptions should act as a guide for the use of different stretching exercises: (a) all athletes have similar flexibility needs; (b) Board Certified Exercise Physiologists know anatomy; (c) most stretching exercises are useless; (d) some stretching exercises are dangerous; (e) flexibility training is focused; (f) flexibility training is progressive; (g) frequency of flexibility training is essential; (h) flexibility training follows a warm-up; (i) flexibility is joint specific; and (j) flexibility training is not about isolation.

All Athletes Have Similar Flexibility Needs

Regardless of the sport, flexibility is important (Box **1**). Whether it is weight training, soccer, gymnastics, or tennis, flexibility is necessary for optimal performance. While other factors may cause problems, such as the failure to train the cardiorespiratory system if you are a track athlete, the lack of flexibility may decrease performance efficiency and may increase the likelihood of an injury (Knapik *et al.* 1992). It is also true that stretching may not prevent an injury in every athlete in every sport (Thacker *et al.* 2004).

Box 1. Flexibility is key to optimal performance.

> "Proper flexibility is necessary for optimal performance. If a joint does not have normal range of motion due to overactive/tight muscles, performance will suffer. For example, if your calf muscles...are tight... your ankle range of motion will be limited. This means you cannot flex your foot enough to get all your power on push off, which would mean a slower race time, a missed rebound, a missed pass, inability to get to the net quick enough, and the list goes on. No matter the sport, proper flexibility is key if you want to perform at your absolute best."
>
> -- Yusuf Boyd, NASM Elite Trainer

What is not well understood is that athletes in different sports do not need to train for increased flexibility using so-called stretching-specific exercises to the sport. In fact, unless there is a prevailing clinical issue, just three flexibility exercises will produce the range of motion required of every athlete. Yes, it is true that some athletes will need to work on their stretching exercises more than other athletes, but they can and should train using the same flexibility program.

The design of the program is essentially the same regardless of the need for more or less range of motion and regardless of the sport. There are no scientific data to support the notion that the soccer player must focus on lower limb exercises while the tennis player must concentrate on upper limb exercises. Both athletes are able to do what they do because of their total body flexibility not because of the range of motion of a specific part. A good flexibility program concentrates first on muscle groups most likely to experience adaptive shortening and then on the most frequently used muscle groups, which may also cause them to shorten.

Knowledge of anatomy provides the understanding that flexibility exercises do not need to be different from one sport to the next in spite of the popularity for sport-specific flexibility training. A highly individualized approach to flexibility training is only necessary for special cases where an obvious musculoskeletal deficiency or injury is limiting the athlete's or client's ability to perform.

Board Certified Exercise Physiologists Know Anatomy

If anything should be apparent to an athlete or a coach today, it is that the number of stretching exercises is very large. The notion that "more is better" is driven by the lack of an understanding of the anatomy of the body. Flexibility training must be built on sound anatomical facts. Only then, can a balanced program in both number and type of exercises result in a significant gain in flexibility.

Without this knowledge, the instructor is likely to encourage the use of a dozen or more stretching exercises. Not only will the stretching session waste time doing useless exercises, it will decrease the benefits of flexibility training. Also, it is likely that dangerous exercises will be introduced. Both can be avoided by doing just "three" exercises to increase the range of motion of all the major muscle groups used by athletes (Box **2**). This is an extremely important point. More is not better. For those who disagree with the statement, it only serves to underline what is already apparent.

Too few instructors, trainers, athletes, coaches, and exercise physiologists have taken the time to study the anatomy of flexibility training. Also, very few college professors have had the opportunity to dissect cadavers to know the specific origins and insertions of the primary extremity muscles. This is a major problem.

Box 2. A fixed stretching routine.

> "As a general rule for stretching and flexibility training, find a small number of good stretches that you can use to form a simple stretching routine and practice them regularly. Don't keep changing the stretches you do whenever you stretch – develop a fixed routine."
>
> -- Idai Makaya

Most Stretching Exercises are Useless

Far too many people fail to realize that the majority of the stretching exercises commonly used are useless. This fact alone is without question a huge surprise to the fitness community and exercise physiologists. The definition for "useless" is based on the following: (a) any stretching exercise used to increase maximal joint range of motion that already has maximal range; and (b) any stretching exercise that results in a meaningless return for the time spent stretching.

Not all flexibility exercises are going to result in an increase in range of motion. This is especially the case if the exercised joints and related muscles are not inflexible in the first place. If such is the case, as is true with neck, wrist, and elbow flexion and extension-hypertension, and knee and ankle flexion and extension, then, the time spent using various stretching exercise could have been better spent with the inflexible muscles.

Why engage in stretching exercises at joints where there are no range of motion limitations? To do so is a waste of time. A track athlete, for example, would not waste training time lifting weights unless a deficiency in muscular strength was evident. Yet, following an injury to the muscles of the posterior leg, an athlete is likely to be encouraged to identify specific weight lifting exercises (perhaps, the calf raise) to rehabilitate the gastrocnemius and soleus complex. Of course the question is this: If the range of motion in the plantar flexors is good, why waste precious training time to stretch the plantar flexors?

On average, it is reasonable to conclude that the shoulder and hip muscles of most athletes and clients are especially tight. The shoulder muscles not only limit the extension and hyperextension (such as the pectoralis major, given its insertion on the lateral lip of the bicipital groove), but also tend to pull the humerus forward and inward. This slightly flexed and inwardly rotated position of the humerus encourages further adaptive shortening. As a result, the upper extremity does not move through extension and hyperextension as it should.

The same sequence of events occurs with the hip flexors, particularly the iliacus and psoas major. After years of sitting with flexed hips and increased anterior convexity of the lumbar spine, both muscles undergo adaptive shortening, which does not allow for a full range of hip hyperextension. Again, the same is true for the hamstrings; a group of muscles that extend the hip and/or flex the knee. When the hamstring muscles shorten from a sedentary existence, they limit hip flexion. Clearly, there are muscles that need flexibility training, and there are muscles that do not need such training. Stretching muscles that already have an adequate range of motion is a waste of time.

Now, as to the second part of the definition, given that the exercise physiologist has selected the stretching exercises, the question becomes, "Are the exercises good or useless (here, we are not considering dangerous)?" A good flexibility exercise is one that allows for optimal benefits in the shortest period of time. In effect, this means that useless exercises result in less than an optimal range in motion with considerable time wasted in the exercise itself. This mistake leaves less time to acquire the range of motion that is needed, and it takes from the actual practice time as well.

An exercise that is good for increasing hip flexion is one in which the athlete or client sits in a straddle position and reaches forward, performing the static stretch method first on one leg, then on the other, and then in the middle. The width of the straddle is increased and/or the duration of the stretch to gradually increased to acquire a greater flexed position. This "good" stretching exercise allows for optimal benefits in a relatively short period of time, particularly in regard to a greater range of motion in the lower back, hamstring, and adductor muscles.

Unfortunately, the naive instructor may have the client stand and lean forward over the thigh to stretch the lower back muscles, gluteal region, and the hamstring muscles. The problem is that this exercise is a balance move in which the person must lean forward hoping not to fall on his or her head. Also, there is no way to systematically ensure that the exercise is producing the desire benefits while the sit-straddle-reach exercise allows for complete control over the force used to stretch the lower back, gluteal, and hamstring muscles (Box **3**). Hence, the athlete can expect and predict as well the desired results.

Box 3. The specificity of stretching.

For a stretching exercise to improve range of motion at specific musculoskeletal joints, it must target specific muscles and provide the appropriate stretch to the muscles to elicit an adaptation to produce an increase in range of motion.

Some Stretching Exercises are Dangerous

The demands of competition and the need to win dictate that most athletes will do what they think is necessary to be number one in their sport. Similarly, many non-athletes are also driven to do and to try whatever to win. The problem is that everyone cannot be a winner in athletic competition. There are too many factors to contend with, many of which the motivated person has little control over (*e.g.,* genetics and differences in neuromuscular abilities). Therefore, from the athlete's perspective, why not try "whatever" and see if it works. This means consuming sports supplements, sports drinks, and trying out training protocols used by the recent winner. Often, it even includes copying another person's warm-up routine (Box **4**) without thinking that some of the flexibility exercises might actually be harmful.

Box 4. Why warm-up?

The warm-up is physical activity that raises the temperature of the muscles, tendons and ligaments. Stretching exercises are best done after the warm-up. Remember, stretching exercises are necessary to train for an increase in flexibility as jogging is necessary to improve the cardiorespiratory system.

Stretching exercises that are risky should be avoided. They are likely to damage muscles and related structures (ligaments, tendons, cartilages, and joint capsule). This is especially the case with athletes who have a limited range of motion to begin with. To perform the exercises in question without the necessary range of motion is foolish.

If a person can perform the exercise safely (*i.e.,* without the likelihood of a negative result), then the exercise is considered a non-dangerous exercise. This is witnessed many times in sports, especially in gymnastics when the lower limbs are placed in positions well beyond what would generally be called a normal range of motion. On the other hand, if the gymnast can perform the front splits without injury, the exercise cannot be classified as "dangerous".

Conversely, where a person is observed to repeatedly attempt an exercise that is not possible because there simply is not an adequate range of motion, the exercise can be classified as dangerous just as running would be dangerous for the heart patient without proper assessment and training. In a sense, dangerous flexibility exercises exist because of the lack of a systematic understanding of anatomy and a well-planned flexibility program (Box **5**).

Box 5. Example of a dangerous stretching exercise.

An excellent example of a potentially dangerous stretching exercise is the hurdler's stretch exercise. The externally rotated leg and, therefore, tibia places an unnecessary stretch on the medial collateral ligament while also placing pressure on the medial meniscus may result in tearing of the cartilage. It may also result in slipping of the knee cap laterally.

Flexibility Training is Focused

The idea that flexibility training is good only if and when it is well balanced is an outdated concept. It is as useless as going to the store to buy a gallon of milk, but before you can do so you have to walk by and give recognition to a dozen or so other foods. Imagine the waste of time when the concern is to get milk and yet because of traditional thinking the immediate need is pushed aside. This is very much the case with flexibility training. Too many unnecessary exercises demand too much time, which is taken from the real issue of working only the muscles that need stretching.

Flexibility training must be focused. Only the muscles that need stretching should be stretched. The athlete's training for an increase in range of motion should lend itself to an enhancement of the joints and muscles limited by immobilization, lack of exercise, and/or injury. In general, the greatest need is increased flexibility of the low back, the gluteal muscles, the hamstrings, and the plantar flexor muscles, regardless of whether it is a class of young gymnasts, a first-year high school track program, a college football or baseball team, or a cardiac rehabilitation program with middle-aged post-myocardial infarction patients.

Flexibility Training is Progressive

The total time spent in actual stretching is in seconds while the workout time for multiple stretches is in minutes. Flexibility training demands a sizable portion of the total workout. That is, if the athlete is interested in developing flexibility and not simply doing a general body warm-up, the time factor is important. After all, changing the structure of the body by way of small micro-adjustments is not something that takes place in one afternoon or even after two or three weeks of commitment. The most effective program requires a disciplined understanding of the anatomy of good *vs.* useless and dangerous flexibility exercises (Box **6**).

Box 6. Flexibility program for heart disease patients.

First, to begin with, be sure to use the "good" stretches three days a week. Second, hold each stretch for 10 seconds to the point of tightness or slight discomfort. Third, repeat each stretch three times. Fourth, remember that stretching is most effective when the muscles are warmed up. Fifth, avoid the useless and the dangerous exercises (regardless of what anyone may say otherwise).

The stretching routine should begin with a 10-second stretch followed by a second set three times a week. After one week, hold the stretch for 20 seconds followed by a second set three times a week. After two weeks, hold the stretch for 30 seconds followed by a second set three times a week. After three weeks, hold the stretch for 30 seconds followed by three sets three times a week. This routine should be used for each of the "three" good stretching exercises.

Frequency of Flexibility Training is Essential

It takes consistency to develop an increase in range of motion. Of course, while it is mandatory for athletes to stretch every day, the non-athlete can afford to engage in a stretching routine two to three times a week. This is a rather major difference between the two, but it is the difference that separates the athlete from the non-athlete.

Athletes need flexibility and, therefore, stretching exercises must be done daily along with their usual athletic training. It is an excellent way to acquire the range of motion necessary to have the freedom to move in sports. Most athletes will do flexibility exercises at the beginning of the workout and other athletes may want to stretch after their workout. The stretching may decrease muscle soreness and induce general body relaxation. If there is a need for individualized stretching exercises (given certain clinical considerations), then time would be allotted for extra sessions either in the morning or late at night just before going to bed.

Non-athletes are less disciplined and, thus their flexibility training is less intense. Stretching three times a week just before each of the three weekly workouts is sufficient to develop and maintain flexibility. Both the workout and the stretching sessions should be evenly spaced over the week. A day between each workout is a good idea to allow the muscles to relax and undergo post-workout adaptations.

During flexibility training the muscle spindles are stimulated to avoid injury (Box 7). Similar to strength development, if more flexibility is desired, either a greater effort is needed during each workout or an increase in the number of sessions per week. But, the effort and frequency must be carried out appropriately. If that is the case, the results (*e.g.,* improvement in muscle function and range of motion as well as improvement in oxygen transport and uptake at the cellular level) are correlated with the progressive application of overload and/or intensity and, therefore, are predictable given a well-planned and disciplined approach.

Box 7. The purpose of the stretch reflex.

When muscles are stretched, receptors within the muscles, known as muscle spindles, are stimulated. A message is sent to the spinal cord that the muscles are being stretched. If the muscles are overstretched or stretched too fast, the spinal cord sends a reflex message to the muscles to contract. This is a basic protective mechanism, referred to as the stretch reflex, to help prevent overstretching and injury.

Flexibility Training Follows a Warm-Up

Stretching exercises should be preceded by a warm-up. Why? Because muscles are somewhat similar to the motor in your car! You would not generally, after getting in your car on a cold morning, cut the motor on and immediately drive away. Most car experts will tell you that the motor should be warmed up so that the oil flows freely to lubricate and protect the working parts. The same is also true for the muscles that need warming up prior to engaging in the flexibility exercises.

An increase in body temperature and a light sweat prior to stretching may help to decrease injury to muscles and connective tissues. While this point bears serious attention, there are several important points to remember (Box **8**). Not all flexibility training sessions must be preceded by the traditional warm-up if the static stretching is initiated very gradually. Although this statement might appear contradictory to earlier comments in this chapter, it is in fact consistent with the idea that a warm-up is important prior to static stretching.

Box 8. Flexibility training is undervalued.

Is it laziness, time restrictions or simply a lack of knowledge about how to train properly for flexibility that people just do not take the time to do so? Whatever the reason might be, it must be corrected. Flexibility training is the most undervalued component of conditioning and yet, muscle tightness is associated with an increased risk of muscle tears. The bottom line is this: Flexibility training is as important as cardiovascular training or muscular strength development. The main point to remember is that regardless of the sport, it is imperative to start with a proper warm-up. Perhaps, it is jogging at a low intensity before sprinting or riding a stationary bike prior to engaging in a more severe form of exercise. Also, stretching the legs and hip muscles will help relax the low back and decrease the likelihood of back pain.

Here, the question is this: Can static stretching be both a warm-up and a means to increasing flexibility without injury? The answer is "yes" if the session begins very slowly. Then, static stretching without jogging in place is the warm-up and can produce sufficient warming of the muscles to produce optimal gains in flexibility. In the case of the gymnast, the warm-up is the stretch of body parts that will be used in the subsequent, more strenuous execution of gymnastic skills. This approach to warming up is sport-specific, which is useful in sports involving the performance of athletic skills (*e.g.*, gymnastics, tennis, basketball, dancing, and figure skating) because it increases the temperature of the body while also allowing for the rehearsal of specific skills.

Flexibility is Joint Specific

Having a range of motion at the hip joints, lower back, and lower extremities to perform a front split on the floor does not mean that the upper limbs will be equally flexible (Box **9**). If they are not as flexible, then, it is essential to be specific when identifying exercises in the flexibility program if flexible upper limbs (such as shoulder flexion, extension, hyperextension, and abduction) are necessary for a good athletic performance.

However, given that all sports require good shoulder, lower back, hip, and ankle flexibility, is it possible to perform one or more stretching exercises to correct the lack of flexibility to allow for normal function? The answer is "yes". Because a lack of normal motion is likely to exists either at the shoulder joint, the low back, hips and knees, or ankles.

Box 9. The exception to the joint specificity principle.

The concept of joint specificity means that a stretching program for the shoulders and lower back will not improve flexibility in any other joints. But, the "exception" is when the stretching exercise accommodates multiple joints (such as the sit-straddle-reach exercise). The exercise stretches the muscles of the lower back, hips, knees, and ankle joints. Also, with the upper limbs in the forward stretched position, the adductor and extensor muscles of the upper limbs are stretched.

Therefore, a sprinter or a gymnast who has tight hamstring muscles and who engages in one or more stretching exercises will eliminate the restriction to move freely. In particular, the gymnast will be able to move with ease in and out of the splits position on the floor. The sprinter will be able to lengthen the stride given less resistance to flex the hips. In terms of a specific need at the shoulders and/or lower body joints, which represents 99% of any flexibility problem, the stretching routine can consists of just "three" exercises.

Flexibility Training is not about Isolation

It is popular to teach that a good flexibility program involves isolating the specific muscles to avoid overcoming the resistance from other muscles. On the surface this thinking makes a lot of sense, but in reality it misses the point. For example, although it is important to stretch the muscles that need stretching, it is clear that more than one muscle group is stretched across several muscle groups. The sit-straddle-reach stretch is a common stretching exercise in gymnastics. In fact, it would be exceptionally difficult to be a gymnast and not engage this exercise on a regular basis.

Gymnasts use the sit-straddle-reach (Box **10**) exercise to stretch the lower back and gluteal muscles, hamstrings (*e.g.,* semitendinosus, semimembranosus, and biceps femoris), adductors (specifically, the adductor longus, adductor brevis, and adductor magnus), and the plantar flexors when the feet are in the dorsi-flexed position. Without question, gymnasts have significantly more range of motion throughout their musculoskeletal system than many other athletes. Thus, the idea that it is better to stretch the posterior aspect of just one thigh before stretching both at the same time is not supported by common practices in gymnastics.

Box 10. The sit-straddle-reach stretch.

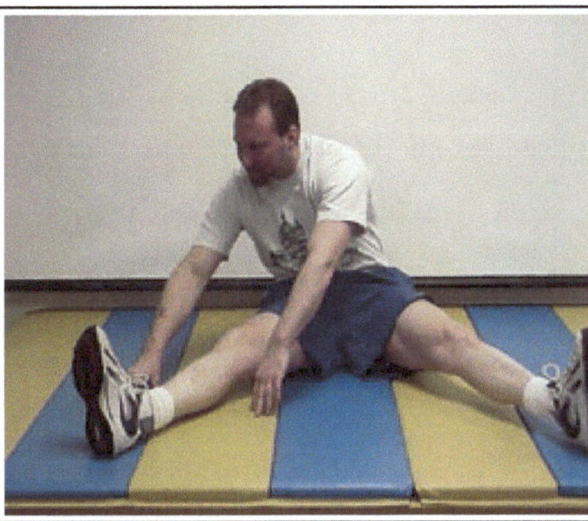

Note that the subject is sitting on the floor with the lower limbs in the abducted position. Depending on the existing range of motion of the adductors, the legs will be either very wide or not so much. This is an excellent stretch of the low back, gluteal, posterior thigh, and adductor muscles. The upper body (from the hips to the shoulders) should be as straight as possible when leaning forwards. Over the course of time, moving the legs wider and wider results in more stretch throughout the body.

Final Thoughts

The assumptions of an anatomical assessment of a flexibility program are not complicated, especially when athletes have similar needs. Therefore, it is not difficult to identified exercises that can be used for all athletes. Good flexibility teachers (such as the Board Certified Exercise Physiologist) know anatomy. Unfortunately, many fitness instructors and trainers who teach stretching routines do not know anatomy. They should be required to learn functional anatomy, including the origins, insertions, and functions of the upper and lower extremities.

The majority of the stretching exercises are useless because they stretch muscles that do not need stretching. Numerous other stretching exercises are dangerous. Without question, several popular stretching exercises increase the risk of injury to joint structures. Flexibility training is focused, progressive, and essential. Athletes and others interested in a greater range of motion cannot turn a blind eye to thinking seriously about stretching, progressing slowly, and staying the course.

Flexibility training follows a warm-up. Optimal benefits occur when the body is properly warmed-up prior to stretching. Flexibility is joint specific. Stretching the lower limbs does not result in benefits in range of motion in the upper limbs. Flexibility training is not about isolating effects. Using an exercise that allows for movement across several joints produces multiple positive effects in range of motion.

GLOSSORY

Anatomy	A branch of science that deals with the form and structure of living organisms.
Flexibility training	A type of training that can improve the range of motion of the muscles and joints.
Hamstrings	Three muscles located on the posterior side of the thigh that extend the hip joint and flex the knee joint.
Muscle spindles	Sensory receptors within a muscle that are sensitive to changes in the length of the muscle.

REFERENCES

Boone, T (2014) *Introduction to exercise physiology.* Jones & Bartlett Publishing, Burlington, Massachusetts.

Knapik, JJ, Jones, BH, Bauman, CL & Harris, JM (1992) Strength, flexibility and athletic injuries. *Sports Med,* 14, 277-88.
[http://dx.doi.org/10.2165/00007256-199214050-00001] [PMID: 1439396]

Thacker, SB, Gilchrist, J, Stroup, DF & Kimsey, CD, Jr (2004) The impact of stretching on sports injury risk: a systematic review of the literature. *Med Sci Sports Exerc,* 36, 371-8.
[http://dx.doi.org/10.1249/01.MSS.0000117134.83018.F7] [PMID: 15076777]

CHAPTER 10

Common Stretching Mistakes

Abstract: Just as the lack of flexibility can lead to muscle and joint injuries and posture issues that influence athletics, health, and wellness, engaging in the common stretching mistakes is a waste of time and a failure to train for an increase in range of motion. It is important to avoid flexibility exercises that are useless. Avoid those that increase the risk of injury, especially the dangerous exercises with questionable value. Only good stretching exercises should be performed by athletes and others. At no time should the joints and muscles be forced into a stretched position. It is always better to engage in a brief, light form of aerobic exercise such as walking or jogging just prior to a commitment to stretching. Also, it is important to recognize the discomfort associated with flexibility training by not over-stretching. When engaged in flexibility training, remember to breathe, to stretch regularly, and to avoid the stretching mistakes.

Keywords: Abduction, Hurdler's stretch, Shoulder extensors, Shoulder flexors, Warm-up.

INTRODUCTION

Flexibility training is not a generalized musculoskeletal warm-up. To improve performance, athletes and others must increase their range of motion across multiple joints. The problem that many coaches, athletes, and others make in training for flexibility is that they fail to understand the infrastructure of the musculoskeletal system. They are not aware that there are useless flexibility exercises, and that some exercises actually increase the chances of an injury. That is why important guidelines exist when engaged in flexibility training.

Avoid Useless Flexibility Exercises

Do not stretch joints and muscles just because someone else is observed doing so. Certain joints and muscles need stretching while others do not. As an example, the

Tommy Boone

shoulder flexors and extensors need stretching while the anterior forearm muscles do not need stretching. To understand which joints and muscles need stretching requires an understanding of why muscles undergo adaptive shortening.

The short answer to adaptive shortening is when the origins and insertions of a muscle group are moved closer together, such as when positioning the wrist in an acute extended position (perhaps, due to an injury). The decreased tension placed on the posterior forearm extensors (Box **1**) will set the stage for a loss of motion.

Box 1. This is a useless stretching exercise.

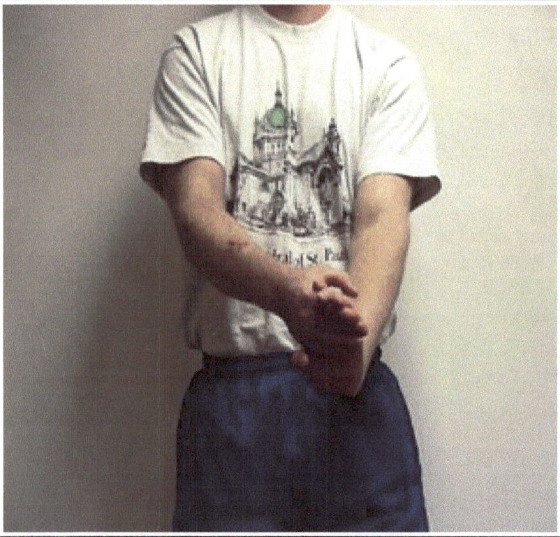

Unless there is an injury or entrapment of the median and ulnar nerves to the forearm flexors, there is little reason to stretch the anterior forearm muscles. To stretch them is to take time away from muscles that need stretching. Thus, this is a useless exercise.

Avoid flexibility exercises that are useless, which is defined in this book as exercises that result in little significant range of motion about a joint(s) because the muscles associated with the joint(s) are not likely to experience adaptive shortening. Aside from the forearm flexors, the quadriceps femoris is another muscle group that athletes and others waste time stretching. Why not use the time to engage in a good stretching exercise?

Avoid the Dangerous Flexibility Exercises

Not all flexibility exercises are safe. Avoid those that increase the risk of injury. They are dangerous and have questionable value. For example, in the track and field sport, there is the running event in which athletes hurdle (jump) numerous obstacles in their path while running at near maximum velocity. The position of one limb that passes over the hurdle is characterized as abducted at the hip while the knee is flexed. The second limb is flexed at the hip with the knee extended over the hurdle. The abducted position of the hip has given rise to the flexibility exercise while sitting called the hurdler's stretch in which one leg is flexed at the knee and laterally rotated. This position places a stretch on the tibia collateral ligament, which is connected to the medial cartilage within the knee joint (Box **2**).

Box 2. The hurdler's stretch is a dangerous stretching exercise.

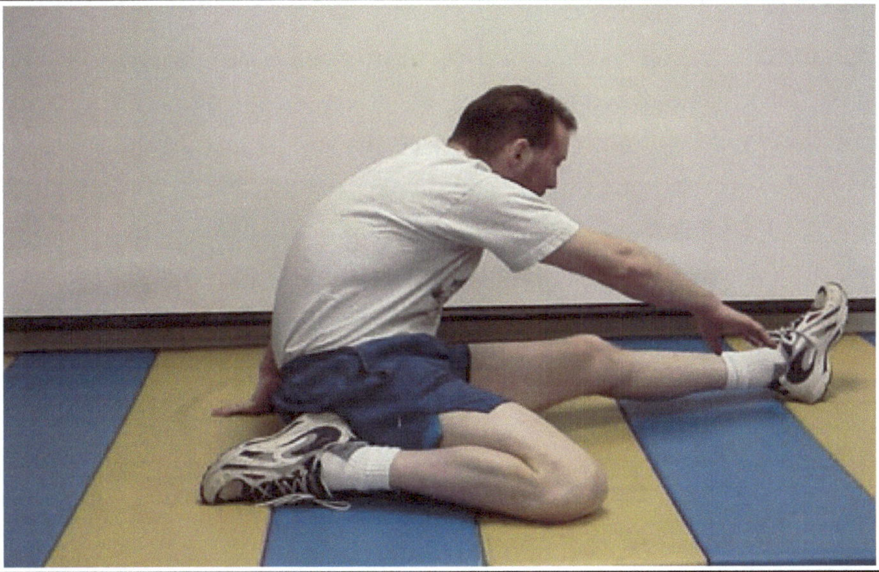

The hurdler's stretch is not the best way to stretch the hamstrings plus it is a very inefficient exercise. The posterior thigh muscles are not stretched since the knee is flexed. So, why is the flexibility exercise still popular? Because hurdlers use the stretch since it approximates the position they are in the air when clearing the hurdles. Aside from this connection with a sport and the fact it has been done forever, there is no logical reason for athletes doing it. Most coaches, exercise physiologists, and athletic trainers recognize the danger of doing this exercise since it also places pressure on the medial meniscus and can cause slippage of the kneecap.

Even more damaging is the same exercise in which athletes are often asked to lay back while the knee is flexed and the foot is alongside the hip region. After doing the opposite side, some trainers encourage the athlete to flex both knees to place the legs alongside the body and then lay back on the floor. The pressure placed on the internal structures of the knees is tremendous. There is additional stress placed on the lower back. By default, the lumbar region of the spine undergoes extreme anterior convexity. This means that the muscles on the back side of the lumbar region are shortened and contracted with the low back acutely arched. It is not a safe position for the spine.

Perform Only Good Flexibility Exercises

Only good stretching exercises should be performed by athletes and others. The definition of "good" is defined as exercises that are most efficient in producing an increase in the range of motion about specific joints. As an example, the sit-straddle-reach exercise with the legs abducted is the most efficient method to increase range of motion of the low back and hamstring muscles than when assuming a similar position while standing (Box **3**). The reason is that the sitting position allows for more control in carrying out the flexed position at the hips with the low back as straight as possible.

Box 3. The sit-straddle-reach is a good stretching exercise.

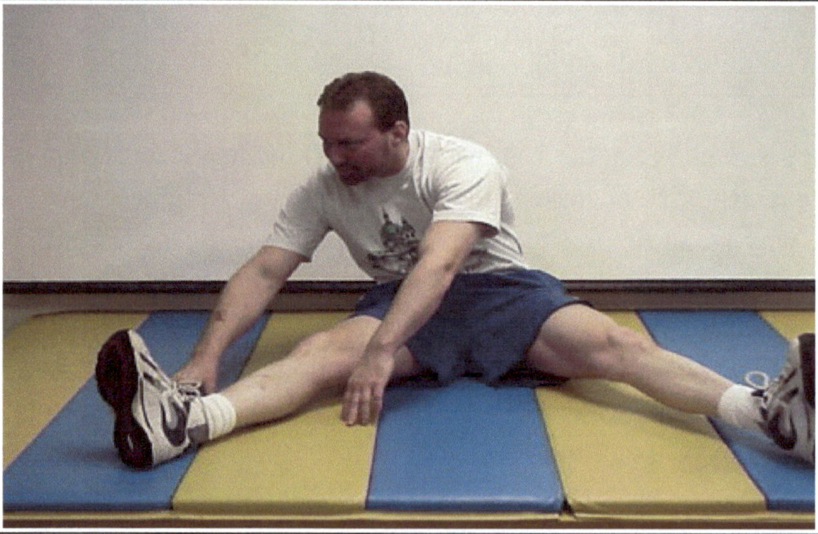

Do not Force Joints and Muscles

At no time should the joints and muscles be forced into a stretched position. The aim is to increase flexibility while avoiding injury. Responding too quickly to a flexibility training program may result in an injury. Expect the benefits to come after weeks or several months of training and not after hours to several days (Box **4**). This thinking applies particularly to muscles and connective tissues that have not been involved in regular exercise.

Box 4. Key points to prevent injury while stretching.

Flexibility is not something general but instead is specific to a particular joint. The resistance to stretching that is offered by the muscles is very much dependent upon the connective tissue. Do not force any flexibility exercise by bouncing or rocking as this may lead to an injury. Flexibility training should take 10 to 15 minutes (or more depending on the athlete or client's history of exercising or clinical condition).

The key is to relax while stretching. The athlete or client should not force him- or herself to touch the toes. Relax as best as possible and breathe while stretching. Breathing is important. One approach is to breathe in at the beginning of the exercise and exhale gradually during the slow stretch and hold. This procedure will promote a relaxed state of mind and body with an increased sense of what is happening to the muscles.

Engage in a Proper Warm-Up

Although infrequently done even by trained athletes, it is always better to engage in a brief, light form of aerobic exercise such as walking or jogging just prior to a concentrated commitment to stretching. Aerobic exercise helps to raise the body's temperature and stimulate the cardiorespiratory system while increasing blood circulation to the working muscles. This helps to decrease muscle stiffness and the likelihood of an injury. Other benefits are include improved health along with an increase in muscle efficiency, a decrease in muscle pulls, an improvement in reaction time, and a decrease in the severity of post-exercise muscle soreness.

Do not Overstretch

Learn to recognize the discomfort associated with flexibility training. No doubt, it will be uncomfortable at first, especially given the tendency to over-stretch. If athletes or clients over-stretch, they will likely be very sore the next day. If that is the case, it is an indication that they should go easier on their stretching by reducing the intensity of the stretches. Overstretching will delay the time it takes to benefit from the "good" stretching exercises. This is because it takes time for the damaged muscles to repair themselves. Naturally, it is important to avoid bouncing during each stretching position and do not expect the desired results too quickly. Do not hold the stretch for an excessive period of time (*e.g.,* 30 seconds is long enough) or stretch too frequently during the initial stages of training.

Perform the Stretch Properly

During the first week, hold the stretch for a short period of time (3 to 5 seconds). Repeat each stretch three times during each of the three sessions (MWF). Later, the duration of the stretch can be increased 10 seconds repeated two times each session. During the third week, the stretch should be 20 seconds each (repeated two times each). By the fourth week, each stretch should be ~30 seconds long. Each stretch should be repeated three times.

Remember that the stretching exercise is not a competition. It must by necessity be individualized (given joint and/or muscle specificity). It is not a complicated understanding that microscopic tearing of muscle fibers and connective tissues results from overstretching. The fastest and most effective way to get hurt is to rush the stretching session. To avoid pain and/or discomfort during stretching, start slow and progress accordingly. The best and safe way to increase flexibility is to perform non-painful stretches, supplemented with relaxation procedures if time permits. Avoid overstretching of the muscles. If the muscles are very sore the day following stretching, do not work as hard at stretching. Lighten up on either the duration or repetition.

Breathing is Important

When engaged in flexibility training, remember to breathe. It helps in relaxing the body to allow the benefits of stretching to be fully realized. So, take a slow and relaxed breath just before the stretch begins and, then, exhale slowly as the muscles are stretched. The inhalation part of the breath cycle should be initiated by the diaphragm muscle more so than the accessory respiratory muscles of the chest (such as the pectoralis major muscles and the sternocleidomastoid muscles in particular).

The exhalation part of the cycle should be natural and slow allowing the air to leave the lungs without forcing it to. Inhalation supplies the lungs with oxygen that diffuses into the pulmonary blood to travel to the heart where it is pumped throughout the body to the muscles. Exhalation ensures that carbon dioxide from cellular metabolism is moved from the pulmonary alveoli to the atmosphere.

Final Thoughts

It is important to point out that some athletes never stretch and they perform well in their sports. They practice their sport, perform daily drills, and compete year after year without experiencing an injury. As they say, "Life is good". A few athletes tend to argue that the only time they were injured in athletics was when they started stretching. Stories like this are primarily the result of athletes and/or coaches failing to understand "how to stretch and why".

Experience supports the belief and the science of stretching that a certain range of motion in the muscles and joints is required for a safe execution of many athletic skills. Gymnastics is a sport that requires a large range of motion throughout the musculoskeletal system. While other sports may not require a lot of flexibility in specific areas of the body, it is always better to train the muscular system for flexibility just as athletes are expected to train for muscle strength and aerobic power (Boone 2016). After all, for the most part, an injury is usually very painful besides being an inconvenience. Hence, when stretching, it is very important to remember the following points:

- Breathing is important
- Perform each of the "three" stretches properly
- Do not overstretch
- Engage in a proper warm-up
- Do not force joints and muscles
- Perform only good flexibility exercises
- Avoid the dangerous flexibility exercises
- Avoid the useless flexibility exercises

GLOSSORY

Abduction	Movement of a limb from the midline of the body.
Hurdler's stretch	The hurdler's stretch exercise mimics the position a hurdler is in as he or she clears the hurdle on the track.
Shoulder extensors	Muscles that are located primarily on the posterior side of the body or shoulder joint (such as the long head of the triceps brachii, posterior deltoid, and latissimus dorsi).
Shoulder flexors	Muscles that are located primarily on the anterior side of the body or shoulder joint (*e.g.*, anterior deltoid, biceps brachii, coracobrachialis, and the clavicular fibers of the pectoralis major).
Warm-up	A brief period of 10 to 15 minutes of preparation (such as engaging in flexibility exercises or a light jog) prior to a performance or an exercise session.

REFERENCES

Boone, T (2014) *Introduction to exercise physiology.* Jones & Bartlett Publishing, Burlington, Massachusetts.

Boone, T (2016) *ASEP's exercise medicine text for exercise physiologists.* Bentham Science Publishing, Beijing, China.
[http://dx.doi.org/10.2174/97816810832161160101]

CHAPTER 11

Good Flexibility Exercises

Abstract: A good flexibility program requires no more than "three" stretching exercises (sit-straddle-reach stretch, shoulder and chest stretch, and the standing hip flexor stretch) to maximize the range of motion of the muscles that undergo adaptive shortening. Increased flexibility in the anterior chest and shoulder muscles, the low back, adductors, hamstrings, and plantar flexor muscles, and the hip flexors, help an athlete or client to engage in athletics or recreational programs, with an increase in skill performance and movement efficiency with less degree of difficulty as compared to earlier musculoskeletal limitations.

Keywords: Athletic performance, Dorsi-flexion, Erector spinae, Hyperextension, Linea aspera, Plantar flexion.

INTRODUCTION

Flexibility training is believed to include many stretching exercises, but such thinking is antiquated and a mistaken reality (McAtee 1993). Books and articles describing dozens upon dozens of stretching exercises abound (Alter 1998). The truth is that a good flexibility program requires no more than "three" exercises to maximize the range of motion of the muscles that undergo adaptive shortening and limit athletic performance, help prevent injury and improve circulation.

Spending a few minutes doing slow, deliberate stretches of 10 or more exercises is very time consuming. Moreover, the time spent in the exercises will do very little to help ensure an increase in range of motion. This means that the exercises are either useless or dangerous. However, it is difficult to accept that with just three "good" stretching exercises, a gymnast can acquire all the range of motion necessary to perform at an elite level is true. Given that this is true for a gymnast,

Tommy Boone

why are other athletes wasting their time doing dozens of useless and dangerous stretching exercises? The only logical answer is that it was the way the athletes were taught by their coaches, trainers, and exercise physiologists.

While what was conveyed to them was perhaps well-intentioned, it is nonetheless unacceptable. That is why the following three flexibility exercises are analyzed anatomically so the reader can conclude for him- or herself the genuine truth of the matter: (a) Sit-Straddle-Reach Stretch; (b) Shoulder and Chest Stretch; and (c) Standing Hip Flexor Stretch.

Sit-Straddle-Reach Stretch

Note that the person is sitting with his legs in a straddle position (Box **1**). The objective is to lean forward first on one thigh for 30 seconds and then on the other thigh for 30 seconds followed by leaning forwards in the middle for 30 seconds. The exercise is repeated three times for ~5 minutes of controlled and focused stretching.

Box 1. The sit-straddle-reach stretch.

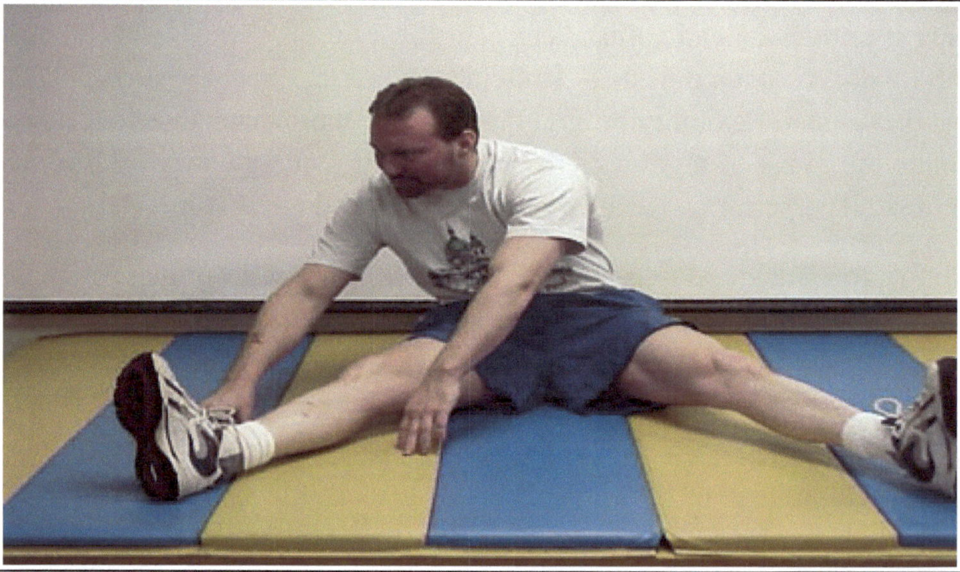

It is a good stretching exercise because it is safe, and because the tension placed on the erector spinae and hamstring muscles is under the athlete's control. Also, when leaning forward, the feet should be in a dorsi-flexed position to help stretch the plantar flexors of the posterior leg. Of course, the idea is to gradually increase the width of the lower limbs, which will place more stress on the adductors of the thighs.

This exercise counteracts the adaptive shortening that occurs with years of sitting and inactivity. The muscles that undergo a decrease in range of motion are the: (a) erector spinae; (b) hamstrings; (c) adductors; and (d) plantar flexors. The arching of the lower back when sitting encourages the low back muscles to shorten, which often results in low back pain (due to the increase in anterior convexity of the spine). The constantly flexed position of the knees with the legs held close together encourages the hamstrings and adductors of the thigh to shorten. The decrease in range of motion of the plantar flexors occurs primarily among women who wear high heeled shoes.

Erector Spinae

The erector spinae (or extensor spinae) is a group of muscles made up of the spinalis (medially), longissimus (center), and iliocostalis (laterally) (Box **2**). Collectively, they arise from a broad and thick tendon that attaches to the crest of the sacrum, the spinous process of the lumbar and the 11th and 12th thoracic vertebrae, and related sacral ligaments. The erector spinae runs along the spine in the thoraco-lumbar and the mid-thoracic area. The muscles are generally the largest in the lumbar region with decreasing size as they move vertically to insert along the vertebrae and ribs. They are innervated by the dorsal rami of the cervical, thoracic, and lumbar spinal nerves. Unilaterally they produce lateral flexion and rotation to the opposite side. Bilateral they help to extend the spine.

The sit-straddle-reach exercise is an excellent way to stretch the erector spinae muscles. To gain full benefit of the stretch, it is important to keep the lumbar and thoracic region as straight as possible when leaning forward. There will be a natural roundness of the mid-thoracic region. Nonetheless, it is best to try to keep the full length of the back straight when flexing at the hips.

Box 2. The deep muscles of the back.

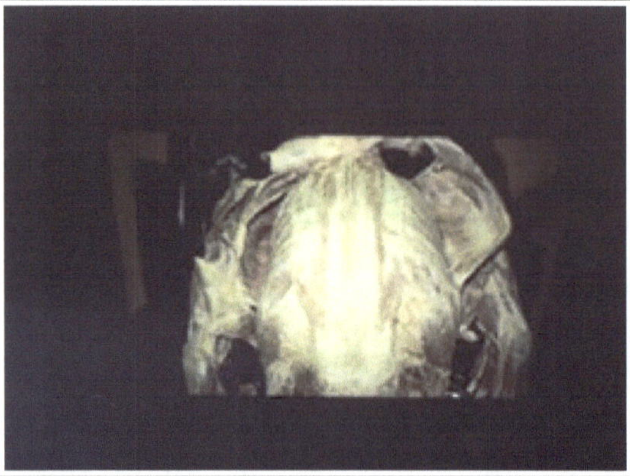

The latissimus dorsi, rhomboid, and trapezius muscles have been released from the respective points of origin, thus allowing the right and left scapula to be moved to the side of the cadaver. This allows for viewing of the erector spinae muscles that run vertically up both sides of the back adjacent to the spinal column. Admittedly, they are not easy to see in the picture. But, there should be the visual impression that they are responsible for positioning the low back and upper thoracis wall in a vertically upright matter.

Hamstrings

The semitendinosus muscle is the first of three hamstring muscles. It arises from the superior lateral surface of the ischial tuberosity to insert on the proximal medial surface (condyle) of the tibia. The signature design of the muscle is its palpable long tendon of insertion. The semitendinosus extends, hyperextends, and adducts the thigh at the hip joint. At the knee joint, it flexes and medially rotates the tibia. The semimembranosus arises from the upper outer quadrant of poster surface of ischial tuberosity. It inserts along with the semitendinosus muscle on the proximal medial surface (condyle) of the tibia (Box **3**).

The third hamstring muscle, the long head of the biceps femoris, arises along with the semitendinosus from the ischial tuberosity to insert on the head of the fibula with a small slip to the lateral condyle of the tibia. All three muscles known as the "hamstrings" are innervated by the medial division of the sciatic nerve. The long head extends, hyperextends, and adductors the thigh at the hip joint while flexing the knee joint. The short head of the biceps femoris arises from the lateral lip of the linea aspera and part of the lateral supracondylar ridge to insert as a common tendon with the long head. The short head is innervated by the lateral division of the sciatic nerve (*i.e.,* the common peroneal nerve). The short head of biceps femoris flexes the knee joint while laterally rotating the tibia with help from the long head. It is the only hamstring muscle innervated by two nerves.

Box 3. The hamstring muscles.

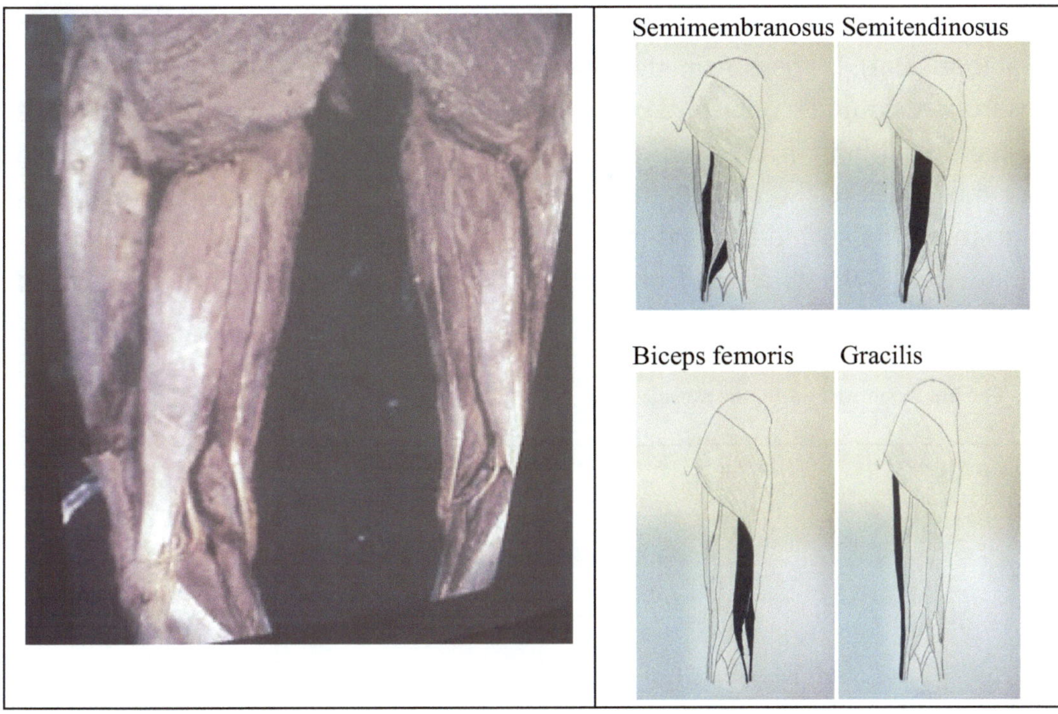

The powerhouse muscle of the posterior thigh that helps the hamstrings at the hip joint is the adductor magnus (vertical fibers). It arises from the lateral aspect of the ischial tuberosity and the inferior surface of the ischium to insert on the full length of the medial lip of the linea aspera, medial supracondylar ridge, and the adductor tubercle. It is a one-joint muscle of the hip joint that is extremely powerful in producing hip extension and hyperextension. It is also an outward rotator of the femur, working with the adductors of the medial thigh.

Adductors

The pectineus muscle (usually identified as the first of the five adductor muscles of the medial thigh) is a flat, quadrangular muscle. It arises from the anterior, superior border of the pubic bone to insert on the pectineal line, which is just inferior to the lessor trochanter of the femur. The pectineus muscle flexes the hip joint, and it can also adduct and externally rotate the thigh. The pectineus is innervated by the femoral nerve, which arises from the anterior horns of spinal segments L2-4 of the lumbar plexus.

The adductor longus (Box **4**) is the second muscle of the medial thigh (*i.e.,* from lateral to medial). It arises from the anterior upper one-half of the symphysis pubis to insert on the middle one-third of the medial lip of the linea aspera. The latter is an osteological bony projection on the dorsal, medial surface of the femur from lessor tuberosity to the medial supracondylar ridge. The adductor longus flexes the hip joint. It also adducts and laterally rotates the thigh. It is innervated by the obturator nerve, which arises from the anterior horns of spinal segments L2-4 of the lumbar plexus.

Box 4. The hip flexor and adductor muscles.

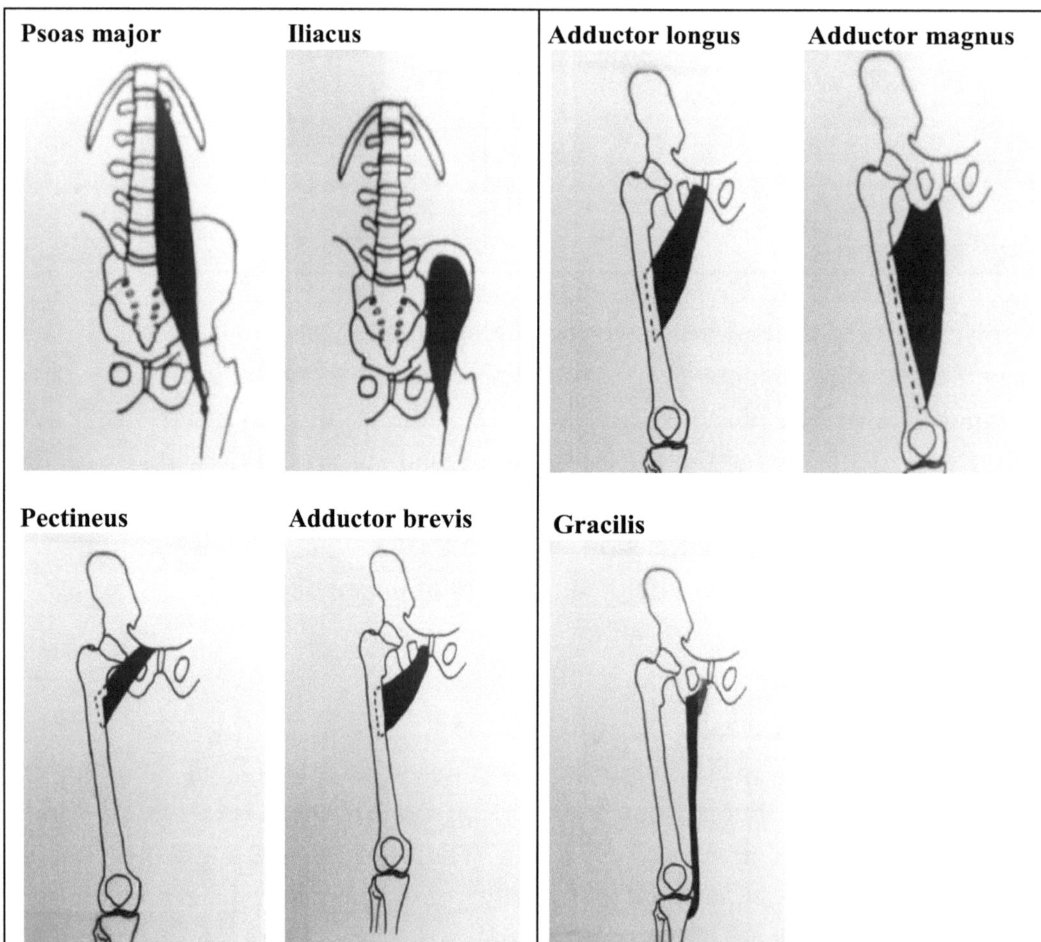

The adductor brevis muscle arises from the inferior border of the pubic bone to insert on the upper one-half of the medial lip of the linea aspera. It flexes the hip joint and adducts and laterally rotates the thigh. Anatomically, from the anterior perspective, the adductor brevis is located posterior to the adductor longus. It is innervated by the obturator nerve.

The anterior fibers of the adductor magnus arises from the inferior lateral border of the pubic bone. Collectively, the fibers inserts on to the upper medial lip of the linea aspera, which approximates the pectineal line. Functionally, it is more like the adductor brevis muscle than the adductor magnus (vertical fibers) muscle. The anterior fibers of the adductor magnus are innervated by the obturator nerve, which arises from the ventral divisions of the 2nd, 3rd, and 4th lumbar nerves in the lumbar plexus.

Plantar Flexors

The least stretched of all the muscles of the low back, hamstrings, adductors, and the muscles that plantar flexor the ankle joint is the latter. There are six plantar flexors in the posterior compartment of the leg and two in the lateral compartment of the leg. The six muscles are innervated by the tibial nerve, which is terminal part of the medial division of the sciatic. The two muscles arising from within the lateral compartment of the leg are innervated by the superficial branch of the common peroneal nerve.

The muscles in the posterior compartment are arranged in two layers, superficial and deep. The superficial layer is made up of three muscles, from superficial to deep, they are: gastrocnemius, plantaris, and soleus. The first two are two-joint muscles. The soleus is a one-joint muscle. The plantaris is the weakest of the plantar flexors while the soleus is the strongest of the three in the superficial layer and the strongest of the eight altogether. The gastrocnemius flexes the knee and plantar flexes the foot. If the knee is flexed, it is not as strong at the ankle joint. The plantaris is 90% tendon and, therefore, without sufficient muscle size to produce a strong force. It is a very weak flexor of the knee and ankle joints.

The gastrocnemius arises from the medial and lateral condyles of the femur to insert onto the dorsal surface of the calcaneus (heel bone). The plantaris arises from the lateral epicondyle of the femur to insert on the more medial side of the dorsal surface of the calcaneus. The soleus arises from the proximal dorsal two-thirds of the fibula and the tibia to insert onto the dorsal surface of the calcaneus. The plantar flexor muscles of the deep layer are commonly identified from medial to lateral. They are the flexor hallucis longus, the tibialis posterior, and the flexor digitorum longus muscles (Box **5**). All three muscles exit the posterior, deep layer of the leg by way of the medial malleolus. The flexor hallucis longus arises from the dorsal distal two-thirds of the fibula to insert *via* the plantar surface of the distal phalanx of digit #1. It plantar flexes and/or inverts the ankle joint while flexing the big toe.

Box 5. The deep plantar flexor muscles of right leg.

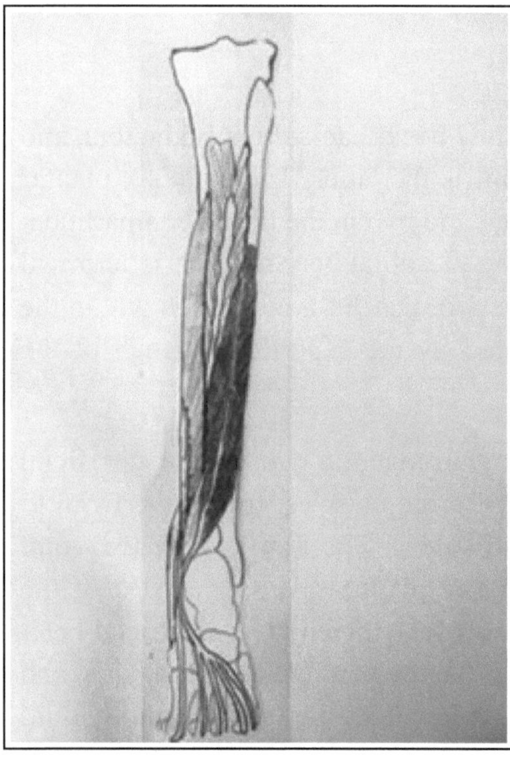

Note that the fibula is on the right side in the illustration. This is a posterior view of the right leg (anatomically speaking, from the knee to the foot). The thigh and leg are referred to as the lower limb.

The deep plantar flexors are identified from lateral to medial (right to left). The first muscle is the flexor hallucis longus. The second muscle is the tibialis posterior, and the third muscle is the flexor digitorum longus. The first and the third muscle insert on the plantar surface of the bases of the distal phalanges. In particular, the third muscle divides into four tendons, which inserts on the plantar surfaces of the distal phalanges of digits 2 to 5. The second muscle lies between muscles 1 and 3. Its insertion is primarily *via* the tuberosity of the navicular.

All three muscles can be stretched when the foot is in the dorsi-flexed position. They are innervated by the tibial nerve.

The tibialis posterior muscle arises from the proximal dorsal two-thirds of the fibula, tibia, and the intervening interosseous membrane to insert by way of the plantar surface of the navicular tuberosity. Its primary responsibility, aside from plantar flexion and inversion, is to support the arch of the foot. The flexor digitorum longus arises from the dorsal distal two-thirds of the tibia and inserts *via* the plantar surfaces of the distal phalanges digits 2-5. It plantar flexes and inverts the ankle joint. It is also the primary flexors of digits 2 through 5.

When the foot is in the dorsi-flexed position (Box **6**) during the standing wall stretch, the position of the foot tends to place a stretch on the these six muscles in the dorsal compartment of the leg, and the two muscles that arise from within the lateral compartment of the leg. The peroneus longus (also known as fibularis longus) arises from the upper one-half of the lateral surface of the fibula and the peroneus brevis (or fibularis brevis) arises from the lower one-half of the lateral surface of the fibula (Nelson & Kokkonen 2007).

Box 6. Dorsi-flexion of the right ankle joint tends to stretch the plantar flexors.

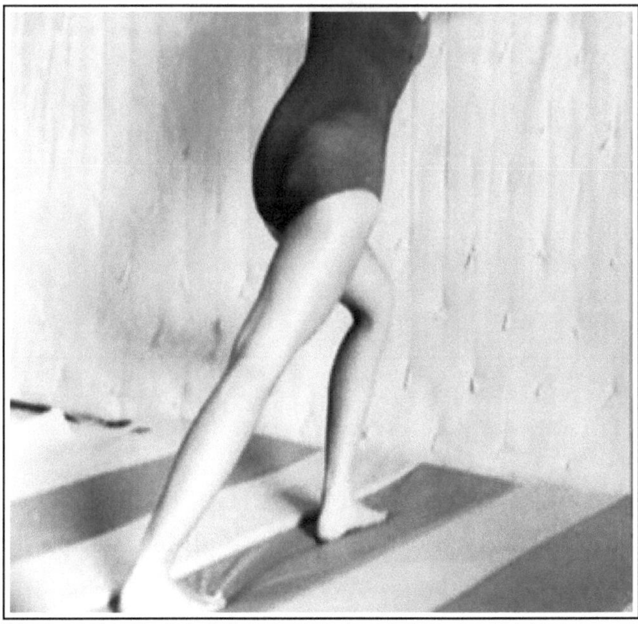

It is important to point out that while this exercise may add some stretch to the plantar flexors, keep in mind that the Achilles tendon (which is known as the calcaneal tendon) is not likely to stretch. It is one of the most frequently injured tendons due to the mechanical loading placed on the tendon.

Interestingly, in 1992, C. Allenmark reported that the calcaneal tendon can withstand repetitive loads equal to ~8 times the body weight.

The peroneus longus ends with a long tendon that runs dorsal to the lateral malleolus to insert on the inferior surfaces of bones on the medial side of the foot, but specifically on the lateral side of the base of the first metatarsal and the lateral-distal end of the medial cuneiform #2. The peroneus brevis muscle also passes dorsal to the lateral malleolus to insert on the dorsal surface of the base of the 5th metatarsal (*i.e.,* the metatarsal that gives rise to the little toe) (Box **7**). Both the peroneus longus and peroneus brevis work with the six primary plantar flexors of the foot and ankle joint (*i.e.,* the gastrocnemius and soleus). Of these two muscles, the soleus is the most powerful plantar flexor since it is a one joint muscle.

Box 7. Peroneus longus and peroneus brevis pass dorsal to lateral malleolus.

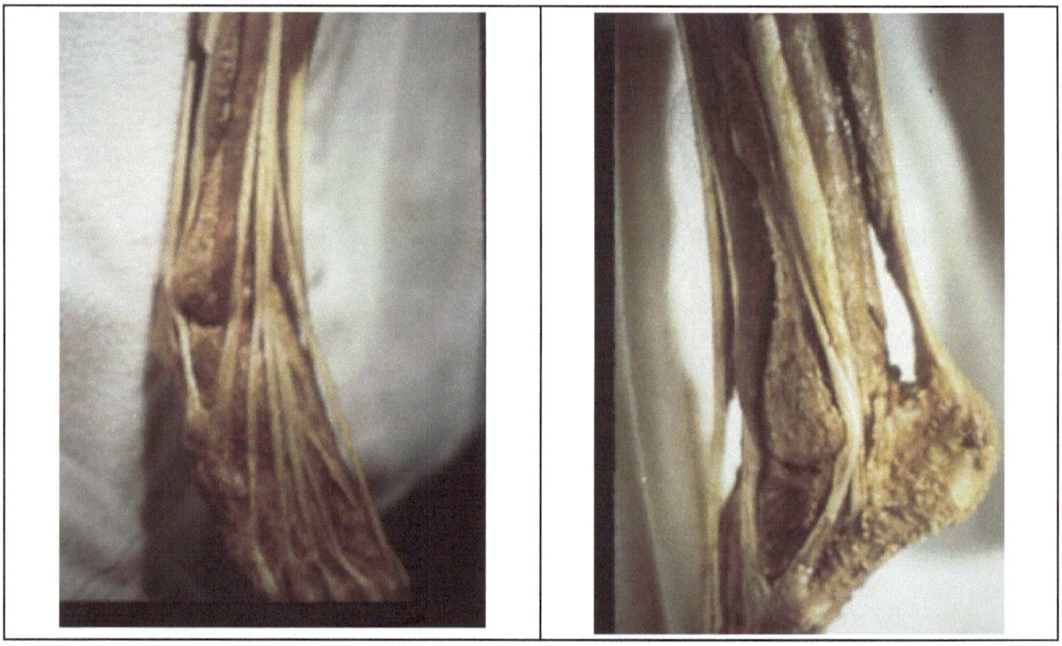

Shoulder and Chest Stretch

The shoulder and chest stretching exercise is important for several reasons. The primary concern is the influence of a sedentary lifestyle on the shoulder and chest muscles that undergo atrophy and loss of strength and endurance. Also, the lack of regular exercise and the predisposition of the upper limbs in the forward position (as when sitting at a desk typing for hours) minimizes the stretch placed on the anterior shoulder and chest muscles. The result is that the loss of a normal range of motion is accompanied by a forward inclination of the shoulders and the tendency to abduct the scapula and round out the upper back.

The shoulder and chest muscles that are stretched during this stretching exercise are the pectoralis major (both the clavicular fibers and the sternocostal fibers), pectoralis minor, anterior deltoid, coracobrachialis, and both the short and long heads of the biceps brachii. Aside from the pectoralis minor that inserts onto the coracoid process and the sternocostal fibers of the pectoralis major, the remaining muscles are the primary should flexors (Box **8**).

Box 8. The shoulder and chest stretch.

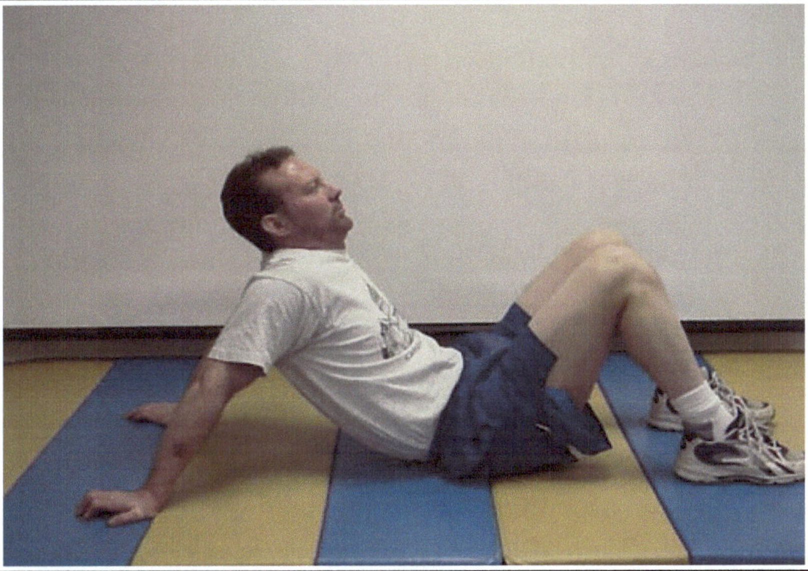

By placing the upper limbs behind the body while sitting and, then, moving the hips forward (as the hips and knees are flexed), the shoulders will undergo hyperextension. This body position will result in a progressive increase in the stretching of the shoulder flexors. This is important because the shortening of the shoulder flexors limits the range of motion of the upper limbs along with the tendency of the shoulders to move forward while the arms inwardly rotate. The newly acquired rounding of the shoulders alters the respiratory activity with a resultant decrease in efficiency of upper extremity.

The clavicular fibers of the pectoralis major arise from the proximal anterior one-half of the clavicle. The fibers converge to insert on the proximal lateral lip of the bicipital groove along with the fibers from the sternal part of the muscle. Both functional parts of the pectoralis major adduct and inwardly rotate the humerus.

The clavicular fibers flex and abduct the shoulder joint while the sternocostal fibers extend and adduct the shoulder joint. The clavicular fibers are innervated by the lateral pectoral nerve (C5, C6) while the sternocostal fibers are innervated by the medial pectoral nerve (C7, C8, T1).

Arising from the anterior distal one-third of the clavicle is the anterior deltoid. The middle deltoid arises from the acromion process of the scapula. The posterior deltoid arises from the spine of the scapula. All three parts of the muscle insert *via* the deltoid tuberosity of the humerus. The anterior deltoid is a shoulder flexor and inward rotator of the humerus. The posterior deltoid is a shoulder extensor and outward rotator of the humerus. The middle deltoid works with both the anterior and posterior deltoid muscles, although it is the strongest of the three in abducting the humerus. The deltoid muscle is innervated by the axillary nerve.

Deep to the pectoralis major and anterior deltoid are two muscles that arise from the coracoid process. They are the coracobrachialis and the short head of the biceps brachii (Box **9**). Both muscles are innervated by the musculocutaneous nerve. They work together to flex, inwardly rotate, and adduct the humerus. When the origin and insertion move close to each other, as in sitting with the arms in front of the chest, the muscles tend to undergo adaptive shortening. To counteract the loss in range of motion the shoulder joints, the shoulder and chest stretch helps to maintain and/or increase the flexibility of the shoulder flexors.

Box 9. Coracobrachialis on the left and the short head of the biceps brachii on the right (in dark on the medial side) and the pectoralis minor arising from the ribs.

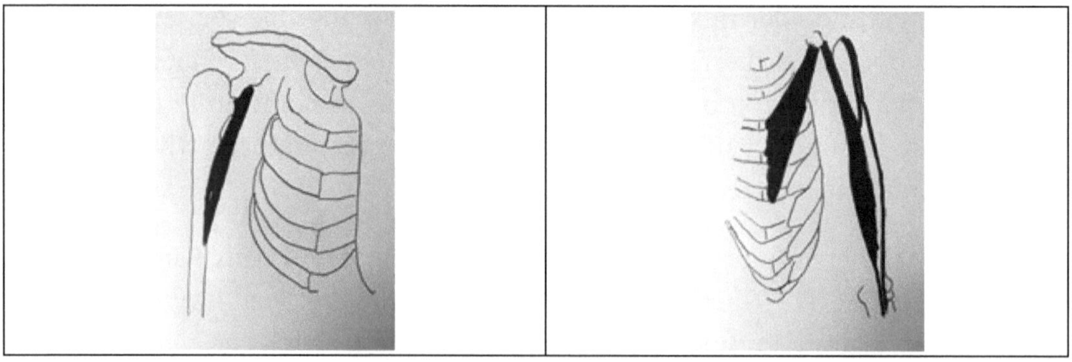

Standing Hip Flexor Stretch

The third exercise of the "good" stretches is the standing hip flexor stretch. One foot is place forward with the knee over the foot. The other foot is place behind the body as illustrated in Box **10**. Note that the upper body is vertical from the head through the hips, which is an important body position. If the chest is positioned forward to a position essentially over the flexed knee, the hip flexors on the straight leg side will not be stretched. After a few seconds of stretching, the back foot is moved a few inches backwards to place a greater stretch on the hip flexors. Then, the exercise is repeated on the other side of the body.

The psoas major, iliacus, tensor fascia latae, gluteus medius (anterior fibers), gluteus minimus (anterior fibers), sartorius, and rectus femoris are the primary muscles stretched during the hip flexor stretch exercise. The secondary muscles stretched are the pectineus, adductor longus, gracilis, adductor brevis, and adductor magnus (anterior fibers). Aside from these muscles acting primarily as hip adductors, they also flex the hip. The hip flexor stretch is an excellent exercise to increase the range of motion of all 12 muscles.

Box 10. The standing hip flexor stretch.

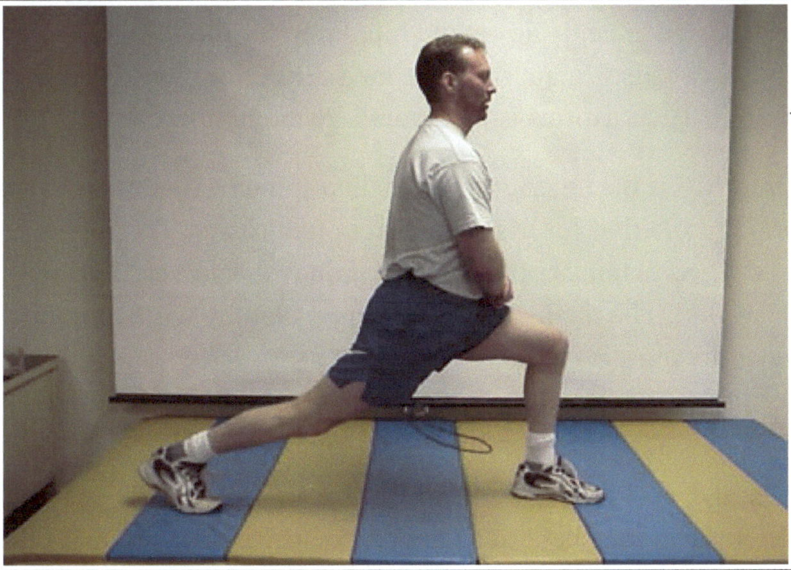

The psoas major muscle arises from the five transverse processes and sides of the lumbar vertebrae to insert along with the iliacus *via* the lesser trochanter. The iliacus arises from the anterior fossa of the ilium. Both muscles are innervated by the femoral nerve of the lumbar plexus. They are also known as the iliopsoas muscle, thus they function as one muscle to flex the hip, adduct the thigh, and outwardly rotate the femur.

The tensor fascia latae arises from the anterior superior iliac spine (ASIS). It inserts *via* the upper one-fourth of the iliotibial tract (also known as the fascia lata). The tensor fascia latae flexes the thigh, internally rotates it, and abducts the lower limb. It is innervated by the superior gluteal nerve, which also innervates the gluteus medius and the gluteus minimus muscles.

The gluteus medius and gluteus minimus originate from the upper posterior surface of the ilium. Aside from their primary action of abduction of the hip joint (along with the tensor fascia latae), the anterior part of each muscle is responsible for flexing the hip joint and inwardly rotating the thigh. The posterior part of both muscles extends the thigh and outwardly rotates the lower limb.

The sartorius also arises from the ASIS. It inserts on the tibia in essentially the same place as the gracilis muscle, although slightly more anterior on the tibia. Like the tensor fascia latae, it flexes the hip, laterally rotates the thigh, and flexes the knee joint. It can also rotate the tibia medially (along with the gracilis) when the knee is flexed. The sartorius is innervated by the femoral nerve.

Just below the ASIS is the anterior inferior iliac spine (AIIS). It is the origin of the rectus femoris muscle that inserts on the tibia tuberosity. The rectus femoris is a hip flexor and knee extensor. It can also abduct the lower limb if the thigh is laterally rotated first. The rectus femoris is innervated by the femoral nerve, which is located under the muscle.

Final Thoughts

Many athletes and non-athletes are not aware that there are "good" flexibility exercises with tremendous benefit to the musculoskeletal system. If they were to engage in just these "three" exercises, athletes would have more time to optimize their full range of motion throughout the body. In fact, it is clear these exercises are sufficient to develop the flexibility that a gymnast needs to perform his or her gymnastic exercises. Given that this is the case with gymnasts as athletes, then, the "sit-straddle-reach stretch, shoulder and chest stretch, and standing hip flexor stretch" would be all that is necessary for all other athletes to maintain their flexibility to execute athletic skills.

GLOSSORY

Dorsi-flexion Occurs when the dorsum (top) of the foot moves toward the anterior surface of the tibia.

Plantar flexion Takes place when foot's dorsum moves away from the anterior surface of the tibia.

Erector spinae A large bundle of muscles that originate near the sacrum and extends vertically up the length of the back.

Hyperextension When extension goes beyond the anatomic reference position.

Linea aspera A prominent ridge running essentially the full length of the posterior aspect of the tibia.

REFERENCES

Allenmark, C (1992) Partial Achilles tendon tears. *Clin Sports Med,* 11, 759-69.
[PMID: 1423696]

Alter, MJ (1998) *Sport stretch: 311 stretches for 41 sports.* Human Kinetics Publishers, Champaign, Illinois.

McAtee, RE (1993) *Facilitated stretching.* Human Kinetics Publishers, Champaign, Illinois.

Nelson, AG & Kokkonen, J (2007) *Stretching anatomy.* Human Kinetics Publishers, Champaign, Illinois.

CHAPTER 12

Useless Flexibility Exercises

Abstract: Useless flexibility exercises are done by athletes, trainers, and other practitioners with the intention of increasing their range of motion. Unfortunately, the time taken to stretch the muscles across specific joints is time wasted that could have been used to obtain benefits from the three good flexibility exercises. This outcome is primarily due to the lack of anatomical knowledge as to whether the range of motion of specific exercises actually produces a significant stretch on the muscles. When an exercise cannot place a stretch on the muscles, it is useless and ineffective and should not be part of the flexibility training program.

Keywords: Anterior forearm flexors, Crooked thinking, Good stretching exercises, Median nerve, Straight thinking.

INTRODUCTION

Although flexibility training is believed to include dozens of different stretching exercises, such thinking is antiquated and anatomically incorrect. Books and articles describing 30 or more stretching exercises abound. Yet, the truth is that an excellent flexibility program requires no more than "three" exercises to maximize the range of motion of the muscles that undergo adaptive shortening and limit athletic performance. However, it is difficult to accept that only three "good" stretching exercises are necessary, it is nonetheless true. Gymnasts can acquire all the range of motion necessary with these three stretches. Given that this is true for a gymnast, why are athletes wasting their time doing useless and/or dangerous stretching exercises? The only logical answer is that it was the way the athletes were taught by their coaches, trainers, and exercise physiologists.

It is unfortunate that there is so little scientific rigor when it comes to doing 10 or

Tommy Boone

more stretches. While many coaches and athletes place a high premium on self-expression, the time spent doing at random exercises will do very little to increase range of motion and the exercise may be dangerous! This is not smart training.

Anterior Forearm Stretch

This is a very common exercise that athletes do. They are under the impression that the exercise produces an increase in the range of motion of the forearm flexors. In general, the muscles of the anterior side of the forearm flex the elbow, wrist, and fingers (Box **1**). They also pronate the hand (*e.g.,* when the elbow is flex at a 90° angle, pronation occurs when the hand is rotated from a palm up position to the down position). The anterior forearm muscles are divided into three layers: superficial, middle, and deep.

Box 1. The anterior forearm stretch exercise.

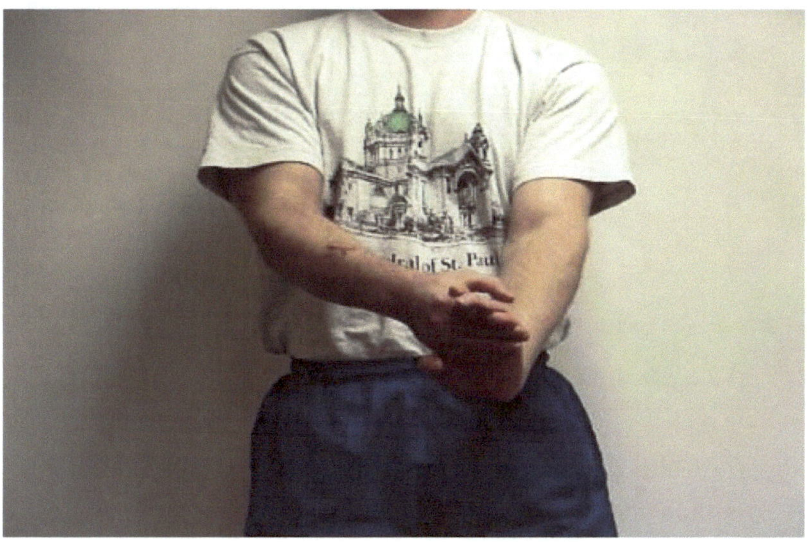

Superficial Layer

With the hand in the supinated position (*i.e.,* palm up when the elbow joint is flexed 90°), the superficial compartment of the anterior forearm consists of the following muscles from lateral to medial: pronator teres, flexor carpi radialis, palmaris longus, and flexor carpi ulnaris. All four muscles originate from the medial epicondyle of the humerus.

The pronator teres originates not only from the medial epicondyle of the humerus, but also from the coronoid process of the ulna (Box **2**). It inserts on to the proximal lateral aspect of the radius. It is innervated by the median nerve, which causes the muscle to contract (*i.e.,* shorten). Given that the points of origin are more stable than the radius, the force of contraction turns the radius medially *via* its long axis. This action on the radius and forearm is called pronation.

Box 2. The forearm muscles of the superficial layer.

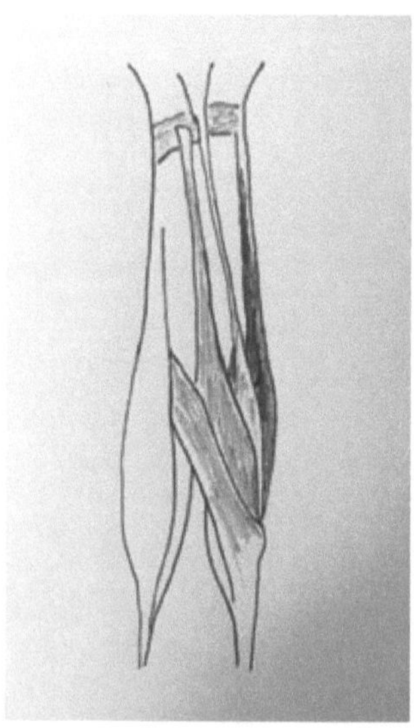

The anatomy illustration of the left forearm is simple but to the point. The four muscles in the superficial layer from lateral to medial are:

1. Pronator teres
2. Flexor carpi radialis
3. Palmaris longus
4. Flexor carpi ulnaris.

While they all originate from the medial epicondyle of the humerus, #**1** does not cross the wrist, #**2** crosses the wrist to attach to the anterior surface of the base of metacarpals 2 and 3, #**3** crosses the wrist to attach to the palmar aponeurosis, and #**4** crosses the wrist to attach to the pisiform and hamate bones of the wrist and then to the base of metacarpal 5 *via* the pisohamate and pisometacarpal ligaments.

Unless there is an injury to the radial nerve on the dorsal side of the forearm that would position the wrist in an acute flexed position, these muscles do not undergo adaptive shortening. Therefore, stretching them is a useless exercise.

As indicated earlier, the flexor carpi radialis arises from the medial epicondyle of the humerus to attach to the proximal anterior surface (*i.e.,* base) of the second and third metacarpals. When the muscle contracts, it flexes the elbow joint and wrist, and abduct the hand at the wrist relative to the forearm. It is innervated by the median nerve. The palmaris longus is the third muscle from lateral to medial in the superficial compartment of the anterior forearm. Interestingly, ~15% of the population does not have this muscle. The primary reason appears to be that the muscle consists of a tendon that is essentially 90% of the muscle's length. The muscle originates from the medial epicondyle and inserts into the palmar aponeurosis of the palm, which is attached to the muscles of the palm. When the palmaris longus muscle contracts, it flexes the elbow joint and wrist. It is innervated by the median nerve.

The fourth muscle in the superficial compartment of the anterior forearm muscles is the flexor carpi ulnaris. It originates from the medial epicondyle, the medial aspect of the olecranon process, and the proximal three-fourths of the dorsal ulnar shaft. The flexor carpi ulnaris inserts on the pisiform and hamate bones with a final distal insertion on the base of the 5th metacarpal. The ulnar nerve is responsible for its contraction, which results in flexion of the elbow joint and flexion and/or adducts of the wrist.

Intermediate Layer

The flexor digitorum superficialis is the only muscle of the intermediate (*i.e.*, middle) layer (Box **3**). It originates from the medial epicondyle of the humerus and the anterior middle one-third of the radius. The muscle gives rise to four tendons that attach to the sides of the middle phalanges of digits 2 through 5. It is innervated by the median nerve. Contraction results in flexion of the elbow, wrist, and metacarpophalangeal joints as well as flexion of the middle phalanges of the fingers at the proximal interphalangeal joints of digits 2 through 5.

Box 3. The flexor digitorum superficialis muscle.

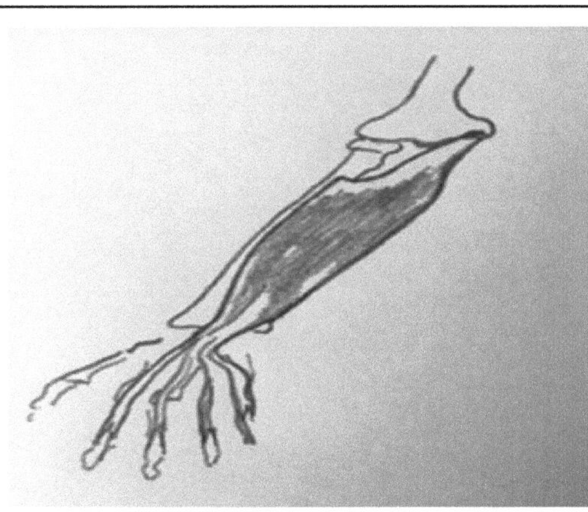

Given the size of the FDS (flexor digitorum superficialis) muscle, it occupies the entire middle layer of the anterior forearm. The muscle functions as though it is actually four muscles. It originates from two major osteological sites (most notably the radius) and inserts on the sides of the middle phalanges of digits 2 to 5.

Deep Layer

There are three muscles in the deep layer of the anterior forearm: flexor digitorum profundus, flexor pollicis longus, and pronator quadratus (Box **4**). The flexor digitorum profundus is deep to the flexor digitorum superficialis. It origin is the proximal anterior-medial two-thirds of the ulna and the interosseous membrane. As the muscle approaches the wrist it splits into four tendons that attach to the anterior surface of the distal phalanges of the digits 2 to 5. When it contracts, the muscle flexes the metacarpophalageal joints (wrist), and distal interphalangeal joints of digits 2 to 5. The ulnar nerve innervates the medial half of the muscle to digits 4 (the ring finger) and 5 (the little finger) while the anterior interosseous branch of the median nerve innervates the lateral half of the muscle to digits 2 (the index finger) and 3 (the middle finger).

With the forearm in the supinated position, the flexor pollicis longus (Box **4**) is lateral to the flexor digitorum profundus. It arises from the anterior surface of the radius and interosseous membrane, and it inserts on the proximal surface of the base of the distal phalanx of digit #1. When the flexor pollicis longus muscle contracts, it flexes the metacarpophalangeal joint and interphalangeal joint of digit 1 (thumb). It is innervated by the anterior interosseous branch of the median nerve.

Box 4. The flexor digitorum profundus muscle (left) and flexor pollicis longus (right).

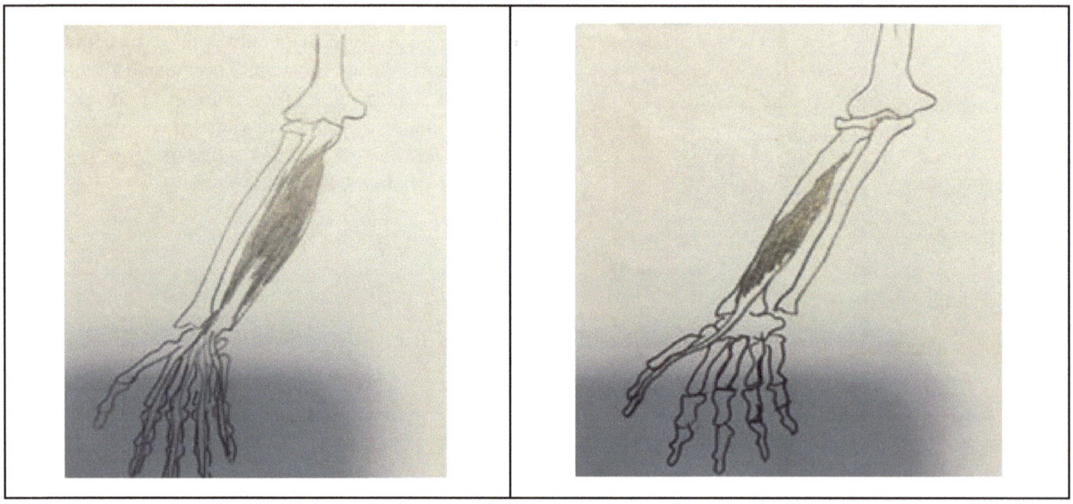

The third muscle of the deep layer is the pronator quadratus. This muscle is actually deep to the flexor digitorum profundus and the flexor pollicis longus that makes it the "fourth" layer of the anterior forearm muscles. But, it is considered as part of the third layer of muscles that make up the anterior forearm (Box **5**). It is the "support" muscle to the pronator teres at the proximal end of the anterior forearm. Thus, both the pronator teres and the square shaped pronator quadratus muscle work together to pronate the forearm and hand. Innervation is by way of the anterior interosseous branch of the median nerve (Drake *et al.* 2005).

Box 5. The pronator quadratus muscle (left & right) and pronator teres (top right).

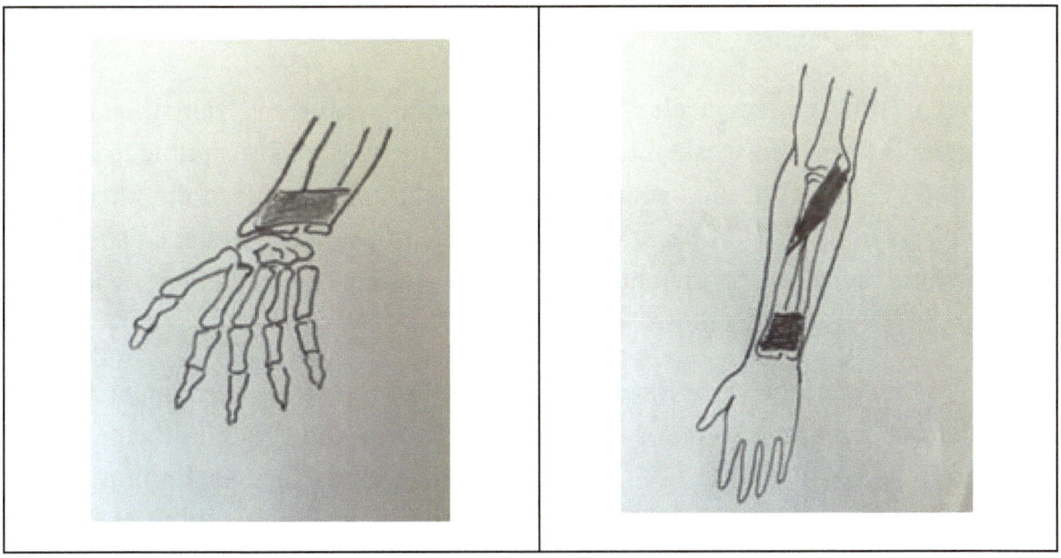

Do the Anterior Forearm Muscles need Stretching?

When most athletes are faced with the decision to stretch the anterior forearm flexors, they do not question whether they need stretching. In almost every instance it is believed that they need stretching. The range of motion at the wrist during flexion is between 60° and 80°. The question is this: What are the factors that might decrease wrist flexion? In short, the primary reason for a decrease in wrist flexion is an injury of the forearm extensor muscles. Here, the point is that a normal range of motion exists between wrist flexion and extension. When the wrist is flexed, the forearm extensors are stretched. Likewise, when the wrist is extended, the forearm flexors are stretched.

If daily motion of flexion and extension of the wrist maintains a normal range of motion, what is the stimulus to shorten the wrist flexors? One possibility may be tendonitis of the forearm flexors and/or inflammation in athletes who perform a lot of repetitive wrist and hand movements (such as rock climbing). Yet, it is interesting that while teaching gymnastics to students and coaching gymnastics for ~15 years none of these conditions was a problem. Instead, muscle imbalance and tendonitis may be an outcome of a work related overuse injury or a sports injury (*e.g.,* Jersey finger). There is also the possibility that a deep cut on the palm side of the forearm, wrist, hand, and fingers can damage the tendons of the anterior forearm flexors.

The point is this. Unless a client, patient, or athlete suffers from rheumatoid arthritis that is known to weaken tendons making them more susceptible to injury, demonstrates pain and/or the inability to bend one or more joints of the fingers, or has numbness of the fingertips, stretching the forearm flexors (and extensors) is a waste of time. This means the anterior forearm stretch exercise is not necessary and, therefore, a useless exercise.

After all, only six of the eight forearm flexors that occupy the three compartments of the anterior forearm pass across the wrist. Moreover, the length of the palmaris longus muscle is ~10% to 15% of the entire muscle-tendon length from origin to insertion, thus any shortening of the muscle would have essentially no effect on not being able to extend the wrist. Of the five anterior forearm flexors remaining, four cross the elbow joint and the wrist.

This means that these muscles (*e.g.,* the flexor carpi radialis, flexor carpi ulnaris, flexor digitorum superficialis, and flexor digitorum profundus) are highly unlikely to undergo adaptive shortening because the elbow joint is constantly extending as is true with wrist extension. Hence, singly or collectively, these actions provide a continued stretching effect on the muscles.

Only one muscle of the eight forearm flexors originates from the anterior forearm itself (*i.e.,* the radius) to cross the wrist. That muscle is the flexor pollicis longus. It is a one-joint muscle that is highly unlikely to experience adaptive shortening unless there is an injury to it. Hence, if the anterior forearm muscles already have a full range of motion, there is no reason to stretch them.

Check this point out for yourself. Stand facing a wall with your arms raised to the horizontal position (in reference to the floor). Place your hands flat on the wall with elbows straight. You should note that essentially the entire surface of the anterior aspect of both hands is fully against the wall. This means the anterior forearm muscles have not undergone adaptive shortening that would otherwise limit wrist extension, and the same procedure can be done in reverse to test the flexibility of the posterior forearm extensor muscles.

Straight Thinking or Crooked Thinking

While our athletic culture places a very high premium on self-expression, the idea that every stretching exercise coexists with anatomic logic is simply wrong. Each person's range of motion is influenced by his or her age, gender, athletic history, work related conditions, and family history. Every athlete or client would have to match up on these factors to assume that all flexibility exercises are good or even safe to perform. The fact is adaptive shortening of the forearm muscles is highly linked to neuromuscular conditions that prevent either side of the forearm from functioning properly, which is not conducive to a person participating in a sports program or someone who is interested in increasing his or her range of motion due to physical inactivity.

If your thinking is straight, the chances of making a wrong decision are greatly decreased. Straight thinking is informative and insightful. It is not a spontaneous reaction to do a stretching exercise simply because you noticed someone else doing it. Otherwise, you are wasting your time, which is more often than not the result of crooked thinking. As an example, the so-called stretching exercises in (Box **6**) are entirely useless. Why are they useless? Because neither exercise can be controlled or practice in such a way as to systematically produce an increase in the range of motion at shoulder joints. Thus, both exercises are a complete waste of time (*i.e.,* they are useless).

Note that flexing the shoulder joint with the right arm and reaching behind the head and neck to touch the left hand positioned behind the back is a movement that is limited by the anatomy of the muscles, tendons, and bones. Similarly, it should be equally clear that the exercise on the right is a useless exercise because there is no way to demonstrate a progressive increase in range of motion as well.

Box 6. Two useless exercises thought to increase shoulder flexibility.

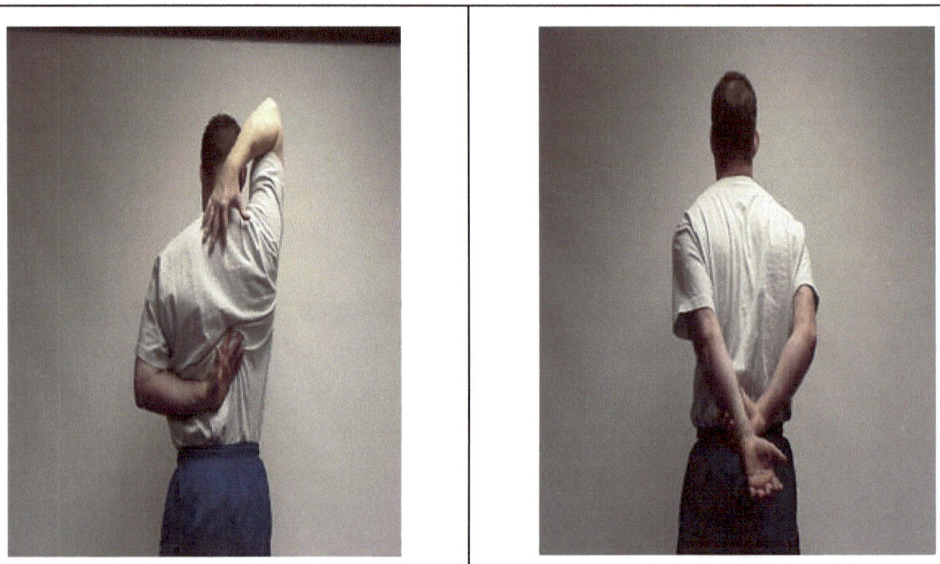

Contrary to the detailed anatomical analysis that was presented with the assertion by many that the anterior forearm muscles must be stretched, it should be obvious that the so-called good stretching exercises in (Box 7) are absolutely useless. There is no way that the exercises are needed by otherwise healthy athletes and/or adults interested in a regular exercise (or athletic) program.

Whether the upper limb was abducted or flexed to position it in the vertical position above the body does not matter. The grasping of the elbow by the right hand with the idea of pulling the vertical limb towards the right is a waste of time. First, if the purpose of the exercise is to stretch the sternal fibers of the pectoralis major, long head of the triceps brachii, and latissimus dorsi muscles, there are much better exercises that can produce positive benefits in range of motion. Second, the fact that the upper extremity is in the vertical position to begin with indicates that the shoulder joint is not limited by the three primary muscles that produce shoulder extension and adduction.

In regards to the exercise illustrated in the right side of (Box **7**), it is a useless because athletes and individuals interested in adopting a less sedentary lifestyle can already do the exercise to maximum. Given that is the case, why do it in the first place?

Box 7. Two useless exercises that are a waste of time.

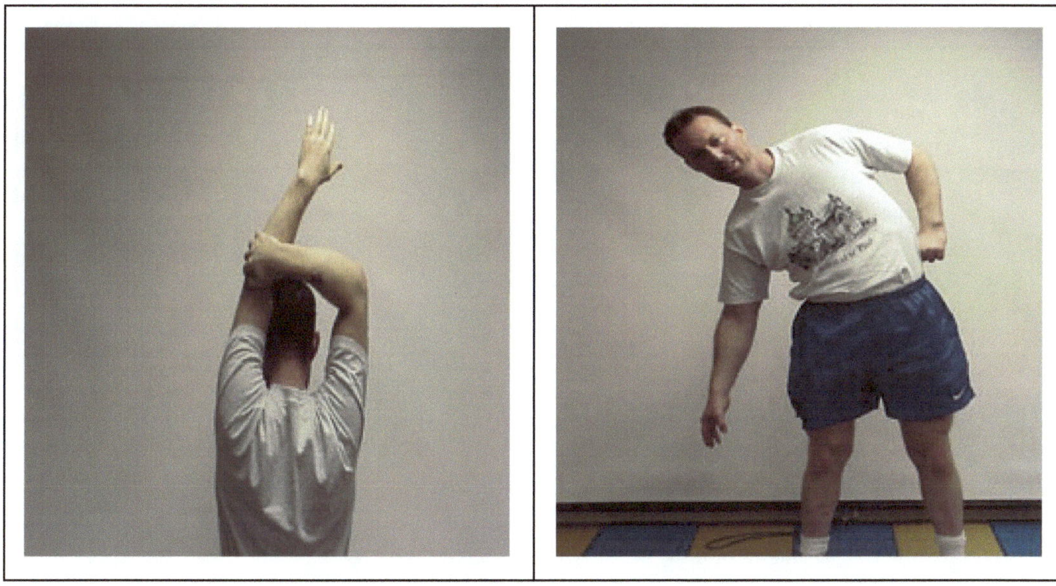

Just because it may feel good does not mean it should be done. Both exercises in (Box **8**) are a good example of this thinking. They are useless because they are not based straight thinking, which would identify the muscles being stretched and how to increase their range of motion over time. With this in mind, the exercise is stretching "what" muscles. Is it the vastus lateralis of the right thigh? If so, isn't the muscle better stretched when the hip is in the extended or hyperextended position while the knee is extended rather than flexed? If the answer is "yes" – then, the exercise is useless.

As to the exercise in the right side of (Box **8**), if the objective is to increase the range of motion of the semitendinosus, semimembranosus, and biceps femoris (*i.e.,* hamstrings) in the left thigh, is there a better way of doing so? The answer is "yes" for a variety of reasons. Truth be known, no one should be surprised that the flexed knee position of the right limb means that the exercise is useless. It is not going to produce a positive benefit. The failure to produce a meaningful increase in flexibility is the primary reason to identify it as useless. In short, it is a waste of time. Why not place the hamstring muscles in both limbs on stretch while stretching one limb more so than the other? The icing on the cake is that the adductors get stretched too.

Box 8. Two so-called flexibility exercises that are meaningless (*i.e.,* useless).

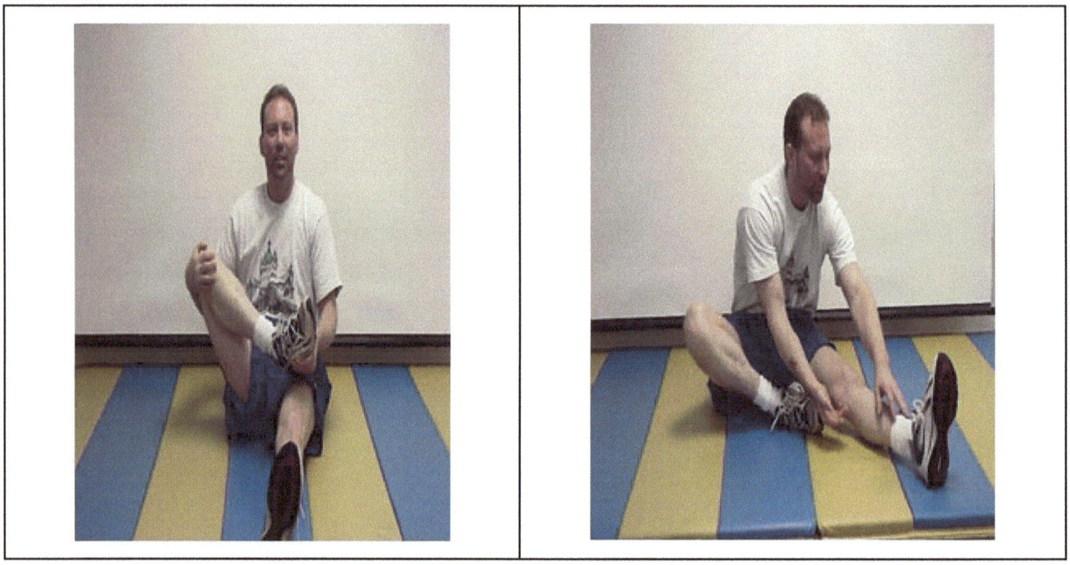

It should also come as no surprise that the exercises in (Box **9**) are useless. In fact, the relevance of flexibility exercises are being undermined and questioned by the simple but fundamentally crooked thinking that these exercises increase range of motion. They do not and yet, there is no shortage of trainers, coaches, athletes, and exercise physiologists who teach these exercises to their clients and friends. Is it possible that they will see what is lacking in these exercises?

Flexibility training is not about just doing any exercise. It is about doing the right exercise. The exercise on the left is useless because the hips are flexed due to the position of the shoulders and upper body. This exercise is suppose to stretch the hip flexors (particularly, the iliopsoas, iliacus, rectus femoris, and sartorious). But, the truth is that none of these muscles is stretched when the hips are flexed. Hence, the exercise is useless and a waste of time.

It is generally understood without a lot of analysis that when clients experience the benefit of flexibility training, their lifestyle changes given that they feel more alive physically. The possession of such insight is freedom to benefit and avoid injury. Yet, it is prerequisite to acknowledge the "good" flexibility exercises from the "useless and/or dangerous" exercises. No one should ignore the useless and potentially dangerous exercise depicted on the right in (Box **9**).

Note that the right knee is fully flexed with the intention to stretch the quadriceps (rectus femoris, vastus medialis, vastus lateralis, and vastus intermedialis). But, the question is this: Are these four muscles (the quadriceps) subject to adaptive shortening that requires stretching? The answer is "no". Moreover, the exercise is not just useless (*i.e.,* a waste of time), it is also potentially very dangerous. The acute knee flexion has the potential to compress the posterior surfaces of the medial and lateral cartilages, which may initiate degenerative changes in each. The menisci are important in that they help to prevent the ends of the bones (femur and tibia) from rubbing against each other.

Box 9. Useless lunge stretch (left) and dangerous hurdler's stretch (right).

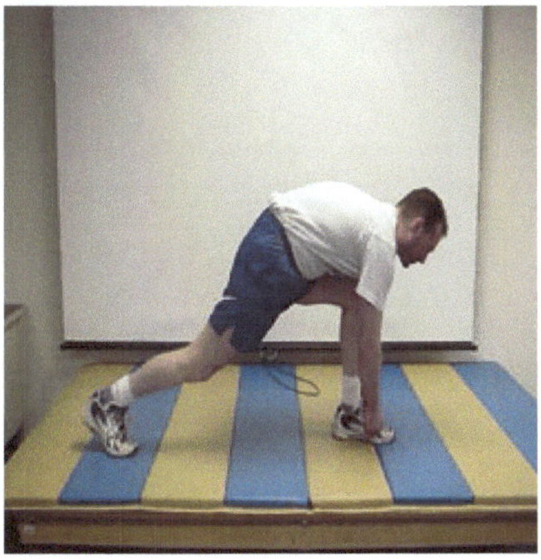

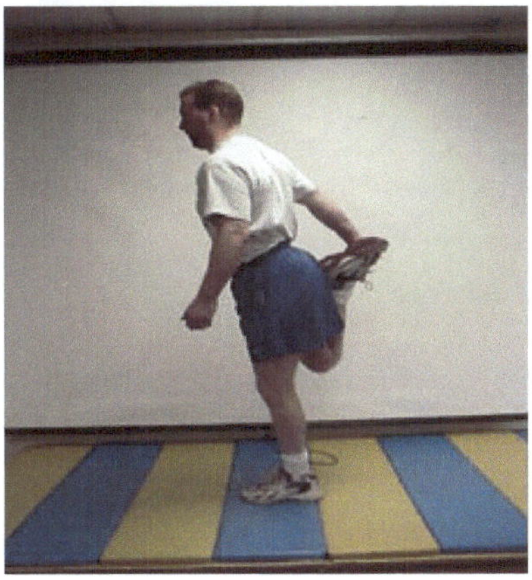

Although there are more useless flexibility exercises than presented here, (Box **10**) presents the final two exercises. Both are rather common and yet, there is no way to ensure an increase in range of motion. It should be obvious that the exercise on the left is useless for stretching the adductor muscles of the thigh (*i.e.,*

the pectineus, gracilis, adductor brevis, adductor longus, and adductor magnus). With the bottom of the feet touching, the knees are pushed downward with the idea that the adductors are stretched.

The exercise is 100% useless and a waste of time. There is no reason to do this exercise. It does not stretch the adductors, which is also true for the exercise to the right of it. This body position is not a stretching exercise, but rather a balance move on the flexed knee side. It is useless, and it is potentially dangerous, given the deep internal pressure on the cartilage of the flexed knee (Boone 2014).

Box 10. Seated butterfly groin stretch (left) and balancing hamstring stretch (right).

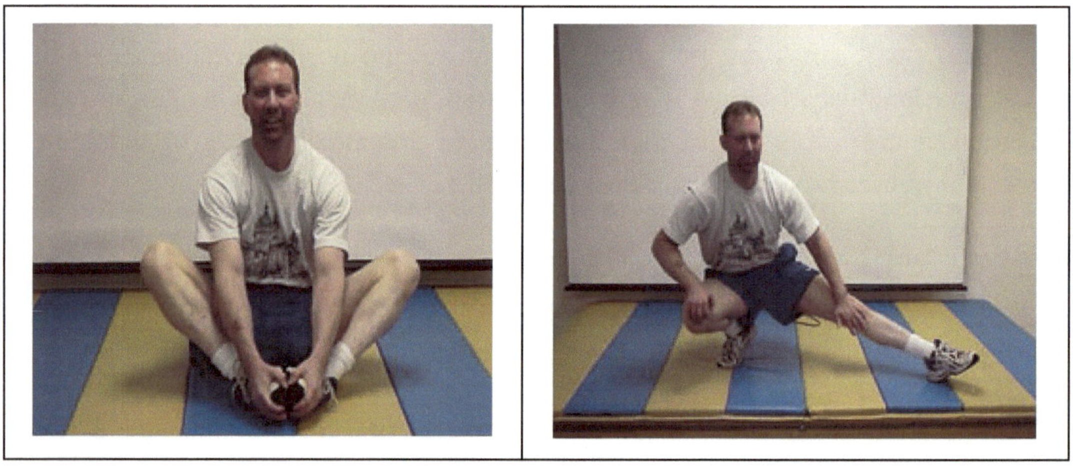

Final Thoughts

You cannot ignore the fact that these useless exercises are rather common among athletes and recreational individuals. Also, unfortunately, there are dozens if not hundreds of equally useless and/or dangerous exercises. The overall result is time lost engaged in the three "good" flexibility exercises. Yet, just look around you and you will see your friends and others engaged in the downward dog stretch, the lying piriformis stretch, the lying spinal twist, the posterior capsular stretch, two legs together hamstring stretch, lying quadriceps stretch, classic standing quadriceps stretch, sitting groin stretch, and the standing calf stretch. If they understood anatomy and embraced even a simplistic appreciation for flexibility guidelines, they would benefit from doing the three "good" flexibility exercises.

Instead, they are missing out on the following:

- An increase in neuromuscular dynamics, efficiency, and coordination specific to better balance and postural control, movement patterns, and the execution of athletic skills.
- A decrease in the risk of musculoskeletal injury.
- An increase in blood flow, oxygen, and nutrients to the muscles.

Today, perhaps more than ever before, society is recognizing that regular exercise is medicine. That is, if exercise is done correctly, it has the power to transform the mind and body. It is for this reason that the commonly practiced flexibility exercises are divided into the good, useless, and dangerous. In doing so, it provides the reader the anatomical and commonsense understanding of a disciplined lifestyle with positive benefits in increased flexibility and decreased negative effects associated with bad practices in sports and fitness training.

GLOSSOARY

Crooked thinking Deception and irrational thinking due to not thinking straight.

Forearm flexors Muscles that occupy three layers of the anterior side of the forearm.

Good stretching exercises Stretching exercises that accomplish what they are intend to do.

Median nerve Originates from the lateral and medial cords of the brachial plexus.

Straight thinking Thinking calmly, clearly, and logically with good judgment.

REFERENCES

Boone, T (2014) *Introduction to exercise physiology.* Jones & Bartlett Publishers, Burlington, Massachusetts.

Boone, T (2015) *Promoting professionalism in exercise physiology: vision, challenges, and opportunities.* The Edwin Mellen Press, Lewiston, New York.

Boone, T (2016) *ASEP's exercise medicine text for exercise physiologists.* Bentham Science Publishing. [http://dx.doi.org/10.2174/97816810832161160101]

Drake, RL, Vogl, W & Mitchell, AW (2005) *Anatomy for students.* Elsevier Inc..

CHAPTER 13

Dangerous Flexibility Exercises

Abstract: A dangerous flexibility program consists of exercises that place unusual and unnecessary stretch and/or force on muscles, joints, and nerves. Many so-called stretching exercises have the potential to do more harm than good. No one should do an exercise that has the potential to result in degenerative changes in joints and nerves over time. Dangerous flexibility exercises that involve placing the head and neck (such as the plough and shoulder stand bicycling), knees (*e.g.,* the deep knee bends and quadriceps stretch), and low back in an awkward or questionable position should be avoided. It is unfortunate that so little credible information is available to athletes, coaches, and individuals interested in flexibility training. The content in this chapter should help lay a solid foundation for thinking straight about which flexibility exercises should be avoided.

Keywords: Controversial flexibility exercises, Dangerous flexibility exercises, Questionable flexibility exercises.

INTRODUCTION

Exercise, whether it is aerobic dance, jogging, or stretching, is filled with the "do this" and "don't do this" type of exercise. In the first place, the "do this exercise" (whatever it may be) and you can expect beneficial results is more often than not highly questionable. If it is the latter case, for example, do not jog in the middle of the day at a temperature of 105° because you can expect a negative result makes sense. But, the certainty should be questioned and/or considered in light of other factors that might also contribute to a benefit or an injury.

When an athlete, college student, or middle-aged person goes to the doctor for an injury from what seems to have resulted from the performance of a skill or, in this case, a flexibility exercise, the verdict is usually a condemnation of the skill or

Tommy Boone

exercise. Seems logical but considering the contribution of other factors (such as inadequate physical preparation or incorrect execution technique) that might have contributed to the result, condemning the exercise may be premature.

Does this mean that there are no dangerous flexibility exercises? The answer is "yes" if the performer's body is capable of adapting to the exercise. The answer is "no" if the performer's body is not capable of adapting to the exercise. Hence, if the person has the prerequisite flexibility to perform a side or front splits, there is no reason to expect an injury from doing either exercise. But, if the person is not ready to do a side splits, then forcing the exercise is very dangerous.

Where there is not a lot of medical evidence to link specific detrimental effects to a particular exercise, then logic (or common sense) must prevail. That is why this book has become so important. There are no absolute answers. There are only possibilities that may or may not surface depending on the appropriateness of the flexibility exercise. For example, a person with a history of back problems should not do exercises that increase the risk of injury to the back. The same is true for a person with knee problems. There is no reason for this person to get into the lotus or the half-lotus position.

Although flexibility training must be tailored to the individual to be safe and effective, the task of doing so is not all that complicated as long as the training program is progressive and guided by common sense. The latter criterion has a lot to do with looking at an exercise and evaluating whether the risks of doing it outweigh the benefits. The potentially dangerous exercises commonly mentioned throughout the scientific literature include the following exercises:

1. Plough
2. Neck circles
3. Bridging
4. Standing toe touch
5. Back hypertension
6. Hurdler's stretch
7. Quadriceps stretch
8. Full squat

The first three exercises address potential problems in the neck region. Exercises four and five are associated with back problems while exercises six, seven, and eight are likely to cause knee problems. In fact, any exercise that produces pain or discomfort or requires unnatural or unusual range of motion should be avoided.

Controversial Neck Exercises

Plough

The plough is performed by lying on the back, raising the lower limbs and hips up and overhead to a point that the feet touch the ground beyond the head (Box **1**). The arms are usually positioned against the ground to keep the body position. The purpose of this exercise is to stretch the back, particularly the mid-thoracic and upper back. The problem with the exercise is that it may result in significant compressive forces on the cervical and upper thoracic vertebrae.

Box 1. The plough stretching exercise.

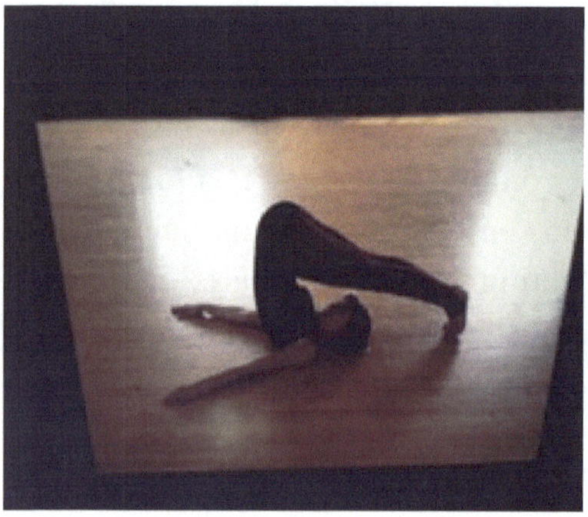

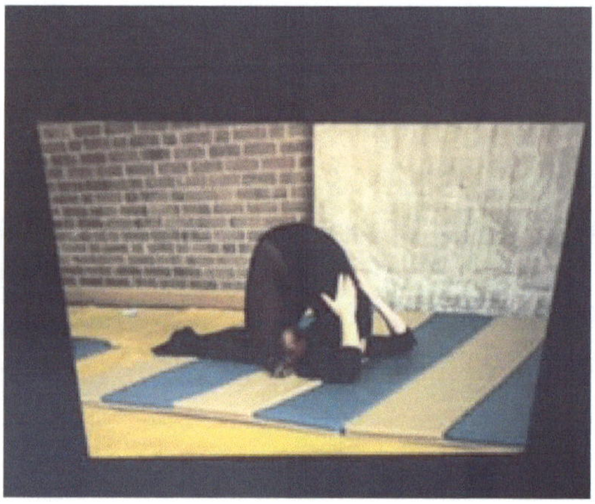

Having coached and taught gymnastics for many years, I can contest to the fact that the plough is not generally a dangerous exercise for the healthy individual or athlete. Of course the position required of the exercise, with increased pressure on the cervical spine, is potentially dangerous for anyone who is overweight and obese. The transfer of body weight over the neck may also be a concern with the elderly. Although they may not have the extra weight to compress the spine, they may have a degenerative joint disease (such as osteoporosis).

Since the plough is a dangerous flexibility exercise for many individuals. What is the Board Certified Exercise Physiologist to do? The answer is simple, given that it has the potential to create a serious problem in the neck region, do not do it and, secondly, it takes time from doing the "good" flexibility exercises. Hence, there is no reason to perform the plough exercise even if the gymnasts, obese subjects, and/or aging clients could do it safely. Why, because the exercise is also useless. Remember if the purpose is to increase back flexibility, there are better, more time efficient flexibility exercises (*e.g.,* the sit-straddle-reach stretch).

Neck Circles

This exercise is considered dangerous for two reasons. First, the hyperextension of the neck may increase pressure on the cervical nerve roots, particularly if degenerative disk disease is present. Second, quick circles of the head and neck may damage the arteries of the neck. The question is this: "Are there sufficient scientific data to warrant exclusion of this exercise (Box **2**) from a flexibility program?" The short answer is "no" but there are concerns. That is why this exercise is listed among the dangerous stretching exercises.

Box 2. The neck circling exercise.

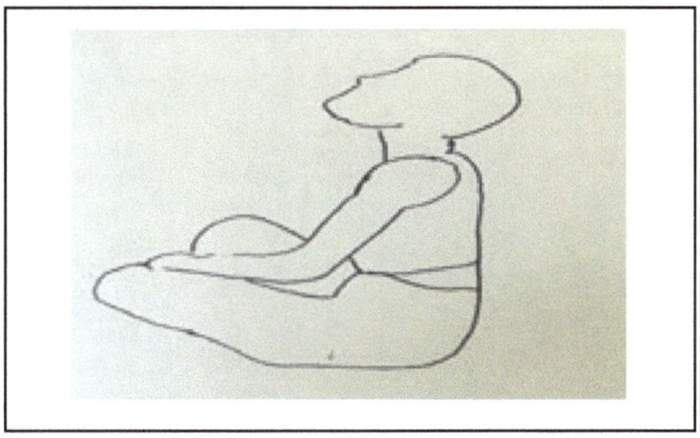

What is important to remember is that the neck muscles do not undergo adaptive shortening. There is little reason to spend time stretching the sternocleidomastoid muscles (neck flexor) or the trapezius muscles (neck extensor and hyperextensor). Even if the exercise is done without problems, it is a moot point if there is no reason to do it. For fitness professionals determined to stretch the neck muscles *via* neck circles, several points should be considered regarding the time involved. In particular, time could be much better spent: (a) stretching the lower back and hamstring muscles; (b) working on the neuromuscular specifics of the sport itself; and (c) substituting a controlled side-to-side and front-to-back motions for the circling motion (that suggests a twisting action at the neck).

Bridging

This exercise is performed by lying on the back with the knees flexed with the palms on the floor by the ears. As the arms and elbows undergo flexion and extension, respectively, the stomach is raised in the air as the hips and back move through extension-hypertension so that the head and feet are supporting the body (Box **3**). Strange as it might be, football players have been seen doing this exercise during the warm-up. It is not a popular or easy to perform exercise and, therefore, few fitness professionals and aerobic dance instructors incorporate it into their routine.

Box 3. The bridge-up stretch.

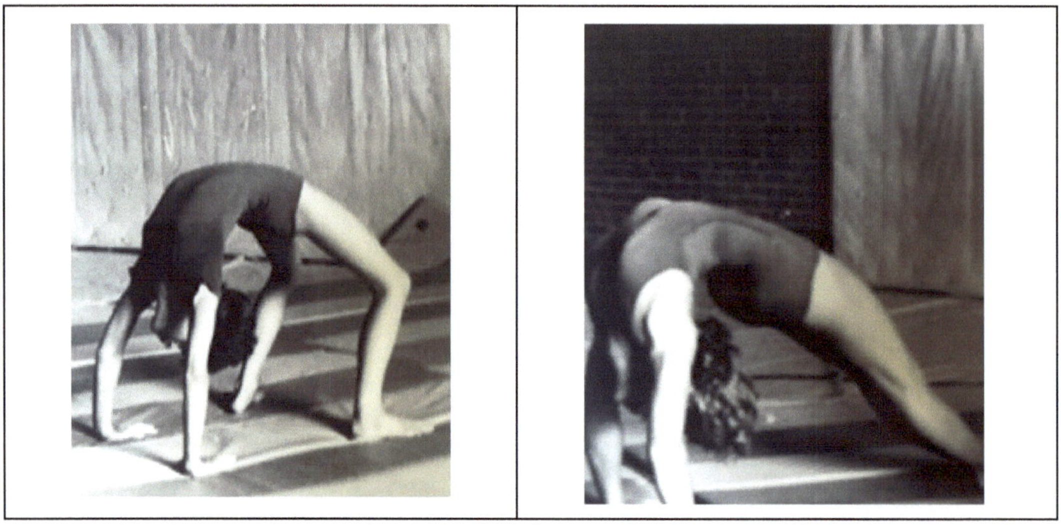

Although the bridge-up exercise is common in gymnastics, it is less so among other athletes. The question is this: "Why would an instructor have his or her client do this exercise (*i.e.,* even if it were possible)?" The exercise places considerable pressure on the back muscles and vertebrae. The problem is that the muscles of the back need to be lengthened (as during hip flexion), not shortened (which is what happens during the hyperextension of the spine). In addition, the hyperextension may increase the likelihood of an unnecessary compression of the intervertebral discs with subsequent damage to the spinal nerves.

Controversial Back Exercises

Standing Toe Touch

Touching the toes from the standing position has been traditionally advocated as a good way to stretch the hamstrings (Box **4**). However, the exercise represents a fine line between being useless and dangerous. Although flexion at the hips allows for some stretching of the hamstring muscles, the stretch occurs while in a somewhat precarious (*i.e.,* balanced) position. There is the tendency to bounce and use gravity to place the chest over the thighs, which results is an increased possibility of compressing the intervertebral discs. The bouncing may also cause the knees to hyperextend, which may be painful. Yet, the compression and pain can be avoided by simply doing the sit-straddle-reach stretch exercise in a much more controlled and efficient body position.

Box 4. The standing toe touch stretch exercise.

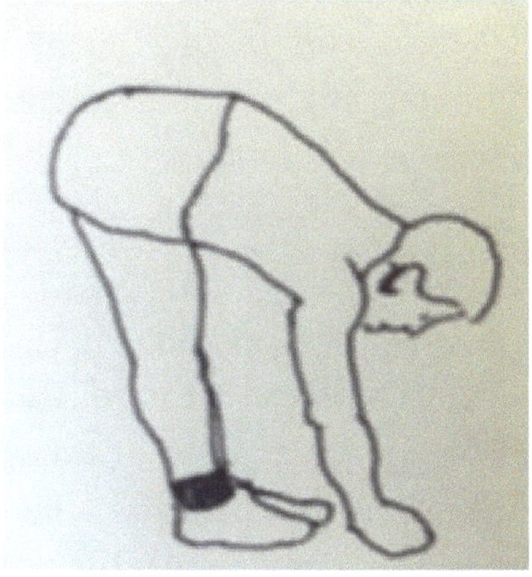

The hamstrings originate from the ischial tuberosity (*i.e.,* the posterior aspect of the pelvis) and insert below the knee joint. With the knees straight, the hamstring muscles are trying to stretch but in reality the tightness pulls the posterior aspect of the pelvis down and back. Given this information as a backdrop, some exercise physiologists believe that the toe touch exercise should not be done because it may allow for an increase in the forward tilt of the pelvis due to the increased capacity of the hamstring muscles to elongate (if that were the case).

In other words, the tension that holds the pelvis in check is reduced somewhat, thus allowing for the undesirable forward tilt with a resulting increase in the anterior convexity of the lumbar spine. This condition of the spine allows for the possibility of an increase in pressure on the posterior region of the lumbar discs. However, the drawback in this thinking is that the increase in flexibility of the hamstrings does not automatically mean that the position of the pelvis will change. Moreover, the tilting of the pelvis forwards or backwards is a function of the strength of the abdominal muscles (and, in particular, the rectus abdominis).

In that muscles experience their greatest lengthening when they are relaxed, the best position to stretch the hamstrings is while sitting in the straddle position with the knee joints extended. Then, the tendency to flex at the hips while leaning over the thighs is less ballistic and more static with a minimum chance of causing a problem. One interesting point, however, is that if an individual realizes that reaching to touch the toes should be done very slowly (although the results will be less positive than when sitting), then may not be a reason to avoid doing the exercise. But, keep in mind that it is an inefficient means of stretching the hamstrings and, in certain situations (such as individuals predisposed to low back problems), it may result in a serious problem.

Back Hyperextension

This exercise is performed in the prone position. It is called the swan exercise, given that the upper and lower limbs are raised from the floor leaving the individual on the stomach (Box **5**). A variation of this exercise is reaching back and holding both ankles (called the cobra position). The full hypertension of the back may cause the soft tissues, articular capsule, ligaments, and disks to become damage. Even when performed as it should be, the risks outweigh the "small to no" benefits to the stretching of the abdominal muscles.

Box 5. The back hypertension exercise.

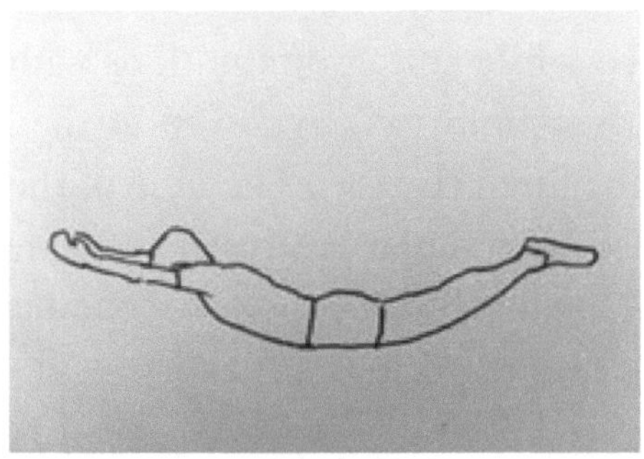

Years ago, it was rather common for the gymnast coach to have a gymnast hold the legs of another gymnast across the parallel bars while he raised and lowered the upper body. Little did the coach know that the exercise was contraindicated in gymnasts with a pre-existing lordotic curve. While the exercise was done to strengthen the back, the problem is that, if the abdominal muscles are weak, the exercise accentuates a pre-existing lordotic curve. Coupled with this result is the fact that the exercise not only strengthens, but tends to shorten the erector spinae muscles of the lower back. The outcome is a coming together of several forces that produce an acute negative lordotic condition (*i.e.,* the exaggeration of an existing anterior convexity of the lumbar spine).

Two variations of this exercise include: (a) the fire hydrant in which one leg is lifted with the knee bent while on the palms and flexed knees; and (b) the donkey kicks in which one leg is flexed and extended several times while on the palms and one flexed knee. Again, the concern is with the movement of the lower limb that results in hyperextension of the lower back. Neither exercise is a stretching exercise. Also, interestingly, even though the fire hydrant and the donkey kicks are two potentially dangerous exercises for the lower back, most healthy young people can do them without hurting themselves. Yet, this does not mean that they should automatically be included in a fitness or flexibility training program. First, the back does not need that kind of exercise (*i.e.,* hyperextension). Second, in doing them, time is taken from doing the "good" stretching exercises.

Controversial Knee Exercises

Hurdler's Stretch

This exercise is performed while sitting on the floor with the lower limbs in the straddle position. One lower limb is then flexed at the knee so that the leg is positioned to the side of the thigh (Box **6**). The tibia of the flexed knee position is generally externally rotated, which places stress on the medial collateral ligament of the knee. Since the ligament is attached to the medial cartilage, the position of the leg tends to place undue stress on the cartilage as well.

If the position of the flexed knee is to enhance the stretch of the hamstrings on that side, it fails 100%. The only way to ensure a satisfactory stretch of a muscle is to avoid reducing the natural length of the muscle before stretching it. Here, we have an exercise in which the hamstrings are allowed to shorten (given the flexed position of the knee) and, therefore, there is no way to effectively stretch the muscle group. By definition, then, the hurdler's stretch is not only dangerous but useless as well.

Box 6. The hurdler's stretch exercise.

<table>
<tr>
<td>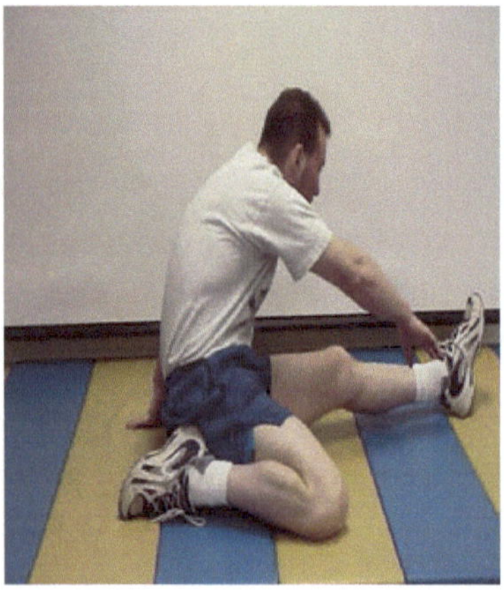</td>
<td>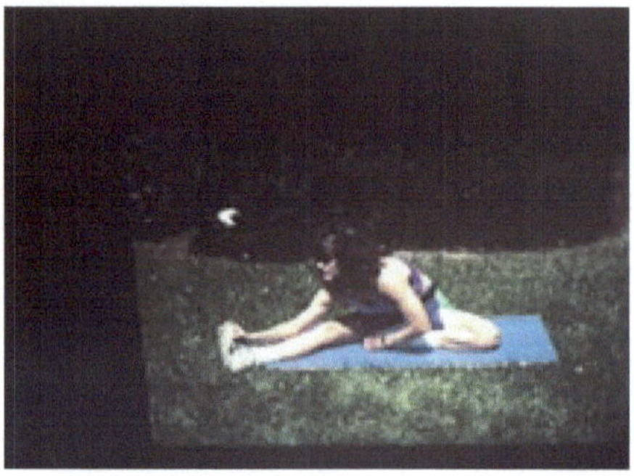
Okay, now the flexed knee is in a better position to avoid injury to ligaments and cartilages. But, it is a "useless" exercise because the position of the flexed left knee distracts tremendously from acquiring a full range of motion throughout the straight right lower limb.</td>
</tr>
</table>

Not only is the exercise in the hurdler's stretch useless, it is potentially dangerous as well. The extreme rotation of the tibia on the femoral condyles may result in an increased laxity of the knee joint and/or disruption of the integrity of the ligamentous structures with possible negative effects on the medial meniscus. Also, in terms of time committed to flexibility training, there is the negative feature of failing to stretch the hamstrings on the flexed knee side.

However, it is well to point out that some individuals can perform the hurdler's stretch (even with both knees flexed) without apparent discomfort or damage. If their knee structure is such that the exercise can be done safely, then the exercise for these individuals is not dangerous. It depends on the individual and, perhaps, many factors yet to be thoroughly understood.

With so many exceptions to the rule, the following question remains: "Should a person incorporate the hurdler's stretch into his or her aerobic dance or fitness program?" The answer is "no" – there is no justification for doing the exercise. There are better, more efficient, and safer exercises to stretch the hamstrings. To do otherwise is neither logical nor professional.

Box 7. The failure to understand anatomy and flexibility training.

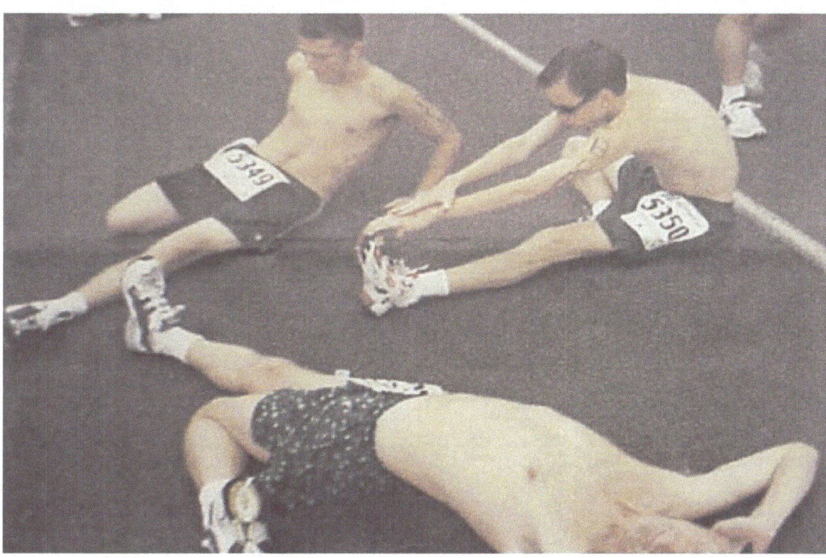

Hence, it is important at this time in the 21st century, given the increased emphasis on exercise medicine, to thoroughly understand that another stretching exercise is just another one to do. It may be good. It may be useless. Or, it may be bad. Now, in regards to Box **7**, breathe in deeply, relax, and expired slowly. Take a look at the following three exercises and think about them.

Full Squat

The full deep knee bend, used sometimes to stretch the quadriceps, is a dangerous exercise due to the tremendous stress on the internal structures of the knee joint. In a nutshell, there is no reason for students or fitness clients do this exercise (Box **8**). If weight lifters or professional athletes consider the exercise as a necessary part of their training, maybe their increased strength will help to stabilize the knee joint and dissipate some of the negative effects. Even though it is clear that some people can do a full squat without joint problems while others cannot, it is always better to be on the safe side. The squat exercise should be performed only to the point that the thighs are parallel with the floor.

Box 8. The full squat exercise.

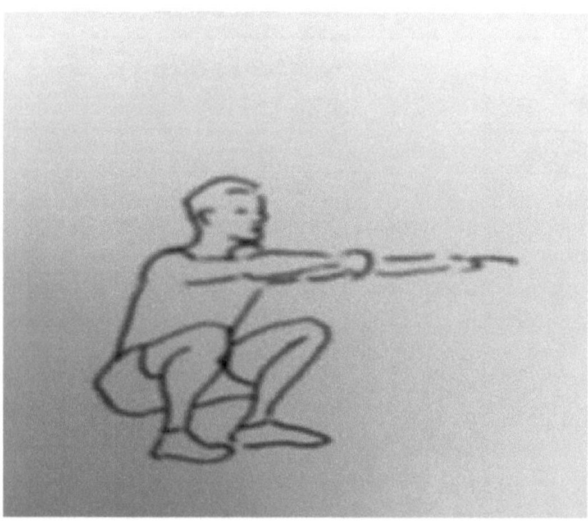

While the full squat is an exercise that may not be good for the knee joints, the primary question is this: "Is it necessary to do the full squat exercise to produce an increase in range of motion of the three one-joint anterior thigh muscles: vastus medialis, vastus intermedius, and vastus lateralis? The short answer is "No". By the way, these muscles do not undergo adaptive shortening. So, why do this exercise if it has the potential for injury to the knee and the muscles do not need stretching in the first place?

If the exercise is done solely as a stretching exercise, it does not make sense. Why, because the quadriceps do not undergo adaptive shortening. Muscles need to be taken off stretch to gradually shorten. Since the quadriceps muscles are always experiencing an elongation of its fibers and connective tissues during knee flexion, it should not be a muscle group that needs a lot of stretching.

In fact, only one of the four anterior thigh muscles is anatomically located to experience some shortening. This muscle is the rectus femoris. It arises from above the hip joint (specifically, the anterior inferior iliac spine and the superior margin of the acetabulum) and inserts below the knee joint on the tibia tuberosity. In the sitting position, the proximal fibers are said to experience some shortening.

However, this does not seem likely since the distal fibers across the knee are under stretch when sitting. In this case, the flexion at the hip and the potential shortening of the muscle is offset by the flexion at the knee joint.

The remaining three muscles (vastus lateralis, vastus medialis, and vastus intermedialis) are one-joint muscles. They are not influenced by what happens at the hip joint. Instead, they are influenced only by the action at the knee joint. As stated earlier, every time the knee is flexed, the muscles crossing the anterior surface of the knee joint are stretched. Therefore, the vastus lateralis, the vastus medialis, and the vastus intermedialis muscles are stretched, which means their natural length is maintained.

Joggers who perform a variation of the full squat by pulling the foot up and behind the hip is not only wasting time doing a useless exercise, but may also hurt the knee joint. Does this mean that all joggers and professional track performers should avoid this exercise? The short answer is "probably not". But, perhaps, most importantly, they should understand that the exercise may threaten the integrity of the knee joint. The payoff is the ability to continue to exercise, and to experience good health and well-being.

Final Thoughts

If a person were to look at the dozens upon dozens of books, articles, and internet pages about flexibility training, it would be hard to conclude there are dangerous stretching exercises. Not surprisingly, the public has come to equate essentially any statement about flexibility as trustworthy. The truth is that most athletes, coaches, personal trainers, and exercise physiologists appear non-interested in the awesome opportunity to think straight about flexibility exercises.

This norm of failing to think straight is problematic. One of the goals of this book is to communicate the truth about flexibility exercises and instill a sense of confidence in the reader that success is possible. It is your choice. Ask yourself, "Would I rather be the one spending my time doing the good stretches or the one continuing to do the useless and/or dangerous stretches?" The truth is this: It makes no sense today wasting precious time engaged in the wrong exercises. Remember, the thinking that resulted in this new way to thinking about flexibility training comes from understanding anatomy. And if you want to be passionate about changing your range of motion limits, you must take anatomy at heart. Tomorrow can happen today if you can visualize anatomy and its foundation to understanding flexibility exercises. The payoff is huge.

You'll never create great flexibility trading time for meaningless exercises. Three stretching exercises are all you need. While they alone can't make you a success, they will not waste your time or slow you down due to a muscle or tendon injury from unsafe stretching. Like the Chinese say, "If you don't change your direction– you're bound to end up where you're headed."

GLOSSORY

Dangerous Involving possible injury or harm.

Meaningless Having no purpose, reason, meaning, or significance.

Questionable Open to uncertainty and doubt.

REFERENCES

Boone, T (2014) *Introduction to exercise physiology.* Jones & Bartlett Publishing, Burlington, Massachusetts.

CHAPTER 14

Historical Issues and Concerns

Abstract: The professional development of exercise physiologists is determined by the quality of their professional thinking, which is in turn determined by the quality of their critical thinking, for critical thinking is the driving force behind professionalism. Without critical thinking, there is little reason to think exercise physiologists are meaningfully interlocked with other healthcare professionals. In fact, it is obvious that all the scientific papers, presentations, and posters by exercise physiologists at national and regional meetings cannot define exercise physiology as a profession. This point is within their understanding if they work at critical thinking as they have taught their students to think scientifically. Yet, many academic exercise physiologists continue to present their scientific papers without internalizing the concepts and principles essential to the professionalism in exercise physiology (*i.e.,* code of ethics, accreditation, and a career specific Board Certification). Despite having the doctorate degree and after teaching years of college and university courses, few professors have the skills to become self-directed, self-monitored, and self-corrective critical thinkers to guide their students' path towards professionalism.

Keywords: Accreditation, ASEP vision, Code of ethics, Exercise physiology, Integrity, Profession, Professional, Professionalism, Traditional thinking.

INTRODUCTION

What constitutes exercise physiology, the issues and pressing concerns of exercise physiologists, and the importance of professional membership? It is not just doing research and publishing. This is the 21st century and many exercise physiologists continue to define exercise physiology as they did in the 20th century. Their failure to get past yesterday's thinking is responsible for the continuation of meaningless academic majors as well as the failure to teach anatomy on the same level as they do exercise physiology (Boone 2010). So much has gone wrong since the 1960s

Tommy Boone

that the traditional thinking associated with getting a college degree is being questioned by students and their parents.

Straight Thinking

While the physical education major was once the primary path for students interested in sports and athletics, that changed as the academic major came under attack for lack of substance. Many departments either dropped the physical education major or changed it to health and kinesiology or exercise science. Others adopted one of 40 different titles. Overall, the change occurred without consistency or a philosophy to ensure academic quality. The well-entrenched failure to think straight has grown in influence, but without professional integrity. Students of exercise science graduate and call themselves exercise physiologists or personal trainers (Ciccolella *et al.* 2008). It is a problem in the United States that stems from decades of exercise physiologists failing to think straight (Box **1**)

Box 1. The importance of thinking straight.

The possibility of thinking differently, changing conditions for students, and attracting colleagues from other fields of work rests entirely with the thoughts of exercise physiologists. Thinking straight is important, as was expressed by Melvin J. Ballard: "Above all else, brethren, let us think straight."

Breakaway thinkers such as the ASEP leaders (American Society of Exercise Physiologists 2016f) and the leadership of the Clinical Exercise Physiology Association (CEPA 2010) assert that the "career needs" of their membership are not being met. If it is true that **what we are to become depends upon what we are thinking**, then, given the smorgasbord of academic degrees students find themselves enrolled in, **the problem is in failing to think straight**. In short, while exercise science graduates may decide to work as a personal trainer, they are not an exercise physiologist unless they pass the "Exercise Physiologist Certified". To think otherwise is wrong and, frankly, it is a very unfortunate outcome of the lack of leadership at the collegiate level that has allowed for the development of a huge list of undergraduate degrees without academic specificity or credibility (Rademacher & Pittsley 2001).

A person who graduates with a nursing degree is rightfully a nurse. Then, too, a person with a degree in physiology is a physiologist. But, clearly, a physiologist is not an exercise physiologist and vice versa. Equally true is the fact that a person with a chemistry degree is not a biologist. The point is a college graduate with a kinesiology or sports science degree is not an exercise physiologist even if he or she has an academic minor in exercise physiology. This thinking applies equally as well to college graduates with a human performance degree. Suppose, for example, if it is true that the kinesiology graduate is a kinesiologist and the sports science major is a sports scientist, it would then make sense that neither is an exercise physiologist (Box **2**).

Box 2. It is all about the title.

> "Be honest with yourself, do you want to be a personal trainer or a Board Certified Exercise Physiologist? Perhaps now is the time to take a closer look at the ASEP Exercise Physiologist Certified (EPC) exam. All I know is, if an exercise science instructor tells you it's not about the title, rest assured that it is all about the title. What's more – if you want to be an exercise physiologist, then you must either graduate with an academic degree in exercise physiology or sit for the EPC exam and pass it. Remember, your future is at stake here… your family's home, your income – your paycheck!"
>
> -- PEPonline
> August 2016

Nothing about this chapter is for the purpose of recrimination of individuals and/or academic departments for what they are. Rather, it is about what can be learned of the mystery of where students, faculty, and exercise physiologists find themselves today? Thoughts have the power to objectify themselves, but a person does not have the right to call him or herself what he or she is not. This is true in law, religion, engineering, occupational therapy, and so on. It should be true in exercise physiology as well.

Students should not be exploited either for the institution's financial incentives or for the politics or business priorities of an organization. And yet, during the past several decades, it has become all too common to encourage students to locate an internship to finalize their academic requirements for graduation. Here is the question: Is it a "good thing" for students? While it appears on the surface to be 100% the right course of action, is it? The truth is this: It is only a good thing up to a point. There isn't any doubt that many students benefit from the hands-on experience that an internship provides. But, unfortunately, it has become too common and expected of many academic majors without an adequate assessment of the assumed benefits. As a result, there is a real concern that students are being taken advantage of by the academic system.

To appreciate the complexity of this all too common requirement, why aren't the departments offering an adequate number of on-campus hands-on laboratory requirements to meet the hands-on skills students need to work safely with clients and patients? Second, it is well known that the internship requirement creates an economic exploitation of the students. Students not only have to pay for the internship tuition dollars, but they must also pay for a place to live (including the travel and the expenses to and from the internship site). It is rare indeed that the student is paid while engaged in the internship. Even then, there is the question of a credible job with a decent salary and health benefits following the completion of all the requirements.

To add insult to injury, students are easily over-powered by the academic process if not dominated by the very teachers and chairpersons who are suppose to be working on their behalf. This is not a trivial point when it comes to the ASEP vision (ASEP 2016g) and goals (ASEP 2016e). The failure of the administrators and faculty to address the quality of career opportunities is a huge reason why the upper administration is responsible for identifying programs that should be dropped from the overall curricular. That is also why, in the near future, students who complete an exercise physiology degree should emerge as professionally competent and aware of the need for a profession-specific organization. As future healthcare professionals (Box **3**), exercise physiology students need a credible evidence-based scientific education to safely prescribe "exercise medicine" to their clients and patients.

Box 3. The definition of a professional.

"A Professional" – Pertaining to a profession, or a calling, conforming to the rules or standards of a profession: following a profession; as, professional knowledge: professional conduct. -- http://www.encyclo.co.uk/webster/P/168

Right now the exercise physiologist's ability to stand apart from the non-exercise physiology major is limited among college graduates. The failure of the academic administration to clean up the non-exercise physiology majors isn't helping. In time, their behavior is likely to be recognized as an unethical turning of a blind eye to the problem. Students and/or their parents should not pay tuition dollars to get a college degree just so college professors can have a job or do research. This means academic exercise physiologists must actively encourage the faculty, department chairs, and/or deans to embrace the ASEP academic exercise physiology standards.

Profession or Semi-Profession

Given Greenwood's (1957) five attributes of a profession (*e.g.,* systematic theory, authority, community sanction, ethical codes, and a culture), exercise physiology is presently more of a semi-profession than a profession. The characterization itself is not demeaning, especially since all professions must evolve from disciplines to semi-professions to professions. Because research is important to exercise physiology, it is more common today to refer to it as a research discipline. Of course this is only appropriate for those with the doctorate degree. And yet, they must learn to appreciate that their professional responsibility is first to their students. It makes little sense for the faculty to spend all their time doing research, publishing scientific papers, attending national meetings, and building their resumes to find that their students cannot find credible employment.

In contrast to the semi-professional status where the students' education is usually a 2-year degree program (Etizioni 1969), Board Certified Exercise Physiologists must have a college degree (ASEP 2016b). Similarly, exercise physiology is a function of a highly specialized body of knowledge, as is evidence by the ASEP accreditation guidelines (ASEP 2016a). After all, given that exercise is medicine, it is important that the prescriptive process is credible and trustworthy. Those who understand this point, especially the Board Certified Exercise Physiologists, are starting their own small healthcare businesses (Ahrens Exercise Physiology 2010). They know what is important, and they are staying the course (Box **4**).

As a healthcare profession, can exercise physiology operate outside of their own professional organization? No, it is clear that they should not. Other healthcare professions do not and, thus it isn't smart to do so. Regular exercise is important, isn't it?

Box 4. Stay the course.

Know what is important and then go after it. Do not let others get you off-track. Talk, write, and live your dream. This is the right path of dealing with apathy. Be positive and stay the course. Or, as John C. Maxwell (2003) said, "The person with a plan, a picture, will go after thoughts that add value to their thinking."

If the answer is "yes" – then, if an exercise physiologist graduates from an ASEP accredited program and, then, sits for the EPC exam, shouldn't the exercise physiologist as a Board Certified professional be recognized as the expert in administering and supervising exercise medicine? The obvious answer is "yes". Is it likely that exercise physiologists will be accepted in society as safe and legitimate if they are not self-regulated by a profession-specific organization? The short answer is "No".

A personal commitment or a calling to exercise physiology means little without dedication to a profession-specific code of ethics and standards of professional practice (Boone 2007a). Hence, in direct opposition to the present-day thinking, the profession of exercise physiology cannot grow if it is always associated with the term exercise science or kinesiology, or if the clinical exercise physiologist in cardiac rehabilitation is always under the supervision of a physical therapist. The Board Certified Exercise Physiologist must be able to make his or her own decisions without external pressure from other professions and/or generic organizations.

The ASEP Organization

Exercise physiologists who support the ASEP professional organization have an interest in exercise medicine. Underpinning this thinking is the familiar concept that speaks to the highest aspirations of a profession (*i.e.,* a profession-specific code of ethics). Competence isn't occasionally argued by the professional organization. It is a constant, and it is not just encouraged but mandated as is true for avoiding conflicts of interest. The bottom line is that all professionals are responsible to a professional practice. That is why the Board Certified Exercise

Physiologists are held accountable to the ASEP standards of professional practice (Boone 2002; Boone 2009).

The ASEP leadership developed the first-ever professional code of ethics for exercise physiologists (ASEP 2016c), developed disciplinary procedures for Board Certified Exercise Physiologists, promoted professionalism, and developed an organizational culture to support commitment to advance exercise physiology.

More non-ASEP exercise physiologists should in good faith seek to help with the change process (*i.e.,* actively support the ASEP leaders). As hard as it is to say, this means on the one hand, dealing with the misinformation as to what is exercise science and exercise physiology and, on the other, doing what is necessary to resolve contradictions arrived at by sheer ignorance or blindness to the reality of reason or evidence.

There isn't any question that organizations are businesses doing what the leaders perceives as their right to maintain an edge over competitors. However, it should be clear that by the pretense of procedural rights that bypass morality by politics, power, and/or greed is an ethical problem that is disturbing and should be rejected (Boone 2007b). Although truths are often uncomfortable realities, professionals must acknowledge that it is not their right to do as they please to maintain status quo. Exercise physiologists must lose something (*e.g.,* the emphasis on research and status) to gain something new, such as credibility and recognition as healthcare professionals. That is why the ASEP leaders believe it is best to give their time, effort, and passion on behalf of the students to help ensure they receive a credible education in return. They believe it is time that the professionalization of exercise physiology begins to take on a larger social and cultural context.

The model of professionalization advanced by ASEP has had much to do with the use of words such as professional, professionalism, professional development, and credibility in exercise physiology (Box **5**). Now, it is fair to say that while ASEP has influenced a major breakthrough in terminology, there is much work to be done. The hypocrisy that surrounds the lack of objectivity in useless academic degree programs must be corrected.

Box 5. Learn to trust yourself.

Without a doubt, leaders often have to make decisions that friends and colleagues are not happy about. Never be afraid to fight for what you believe is important, especially when it helps others. After all, as Vince Lombardi, NFL Hall of Fame Coach said, "The joy is in creating, not maintaining."

One would think that the academic exercise physiologists (especially those who earned the doctorate degree in the 60s, 70s, and 80s) are more aware of the lack of professionalization in exercise physiology. But, unfortunately, many are simply indifferent to doing anything about it. In fact, it is a cop out to argue that they were too inextricably bound up with transitioning from physical education to that of a "scientist" way of thinking to have not known what was necessary to do. Not knowing that they should speak to, engage in, and develop the professional transformation that has been so evident with other professions (such as physical therapy and athletic training) is to miss the point of professional advancement. It seems that there can be only one conclusion. Is it not possible that the absence of discussions pertaining to professionalism while being physical educators left them without knowledge of the understanding and purpose of professionalism and credibility?

Bruhn (2001) said, "Professionalism is an attitude, a state of mind." What is the exercise physiologist's attitude towards professionalism? It is important to know the exercise physiologist's state of mind. Then, one could answer why exercise physiologists are not relying on the ASEP code of ethics when they provide professional services. Does it have something to do with their image of exercise physiology as a research discipline and not as a healthcare profession? Why are exercise physiologists reluctant to pursue ASEP academic accreditation and Board Certification as a professional development opportunity within exercise physiology? Where is their sense of pride when it comes to supporting exercise physiology? Is this professional behavior, which raises the following questions? Why aren't colleagues more civil with each other? Why aren't they more ethical, honest, and consistent communicators with each other? Why aren't they more accountable, collaborative, forgiving, current, and involved in developing exercise physiology as a healthcare profession?

The ASEP Definition of Exercise Physiology

The ASEP leaders understood early on that a lot of confusion centered on "who is" and "who isn't an exercise physiologist". The only semi-universal definition of exercise physiology within academia for the past several decades is whether a person has the doctorate degree. As strange as it might sound, there are many doctorate-prepared exercise physiologists who do not want a recent college graduate with a degree in exercise physiology call him- or herself an exercise physiologist. Fortunately, such thinking is changing. One only has to look at the ASEP definition of an exercise physiologist (Box **6**) to see how the ASEP leadership and organizational thinking differ from the thinking of exercise physiologists who are members of generic organizations (ASEP 2016d).

Box 6. The ASEP definition of an exercise physiologist.

"**Exercise physiologist** is a person who has an academic degree in exercise physiology, or who is certified by ASEP to practice exercise physiology [*via* the Exercise Physiologist Certified exam (EPC)], or who has a doctorate degree with an academic degree or emphasis in exercise physiology from an accredited college or university."

The ASEP definition is straight to the point. If a person graduates with a degree in exercise physiology, he or she is an exercise physiologist. However, from the ASEP perspective, that person still needs to sit for the Board Certification to practice exercise physiology. This doesn't mean that the non-exercise physiology college graduate by degree title per se cannot become an exercise physiologist. A person who graduates with an exercise science (or similar degree) but who has taken a certain number of exercise physiology listed courses and who has had sufficient laboratory experiences can sit for the exam to earn the professional title Exercise Physiologist. This latter track is likely to remain available to college graduates for several decades.

Final Thoughts

To emphasize the original point (*i.e.,* the importance of the degree title), a person who graduates with a college degree in exercise science or kinesiology or one of the several dozen similar academic degrees is not an exercise physiologist. This is true regardless of whether the person is hired as an exercise physiologist or not.

Neither the employer nor the job title defines who is an exercise physiologist.

In other words, it doesn't matter if the employer hires a nurse as a lawyer. A person without a law degree is not a lawyer, and even that person must pass the bar exam to practice law. This thinking isn't complicated, yet the failed rhetoric of sports medicine and exercise science is all too common in exercise science and, yes, exercise physiology as well. This has led to a great misunderstanding of the academic differences between the two degree titles. It is unfortunately but true that the preoccupation with exercise science at the expense of professionalism in exercise physiology has eroded the exercise physiology education (Box 7).

Box 7. The "typical" exercise physiology curriculum.

Today's exercise physiology curriculum is less credible than desired. In particular, there are obvious problems with the exercise physiology academic curriculum and degree program that fails to emphasize professionalism, credibility, career-specific employment and, yes, anatomy!

GLOSSORY

Accreditation The process of granting professional recognition to an academic institution that maintains specific academic and professional standards.

ASEP vision As a national non-profit professional organization, the American Society of Exercise Physiologists (ASEP) is committed to the advancement of exercise physiologists as healthcare professionals. Founded in 1997 in the state of Minnesota, the Society provides a forum for leadership and exchange of information to stimulate discussion and collaboration among exercise physiologists active in all aspects of the profession. The Society works to set standards for exercise physiologists through ASEP-approved curricula in universities and colleges in the United States (www.asep.org/index.php/about-asep/).

Code of ethics Ethical principles and guidelines based on the organization's core values and the standards to which the professional is held.

Integrity The quality of being honest, fair, and having strong moral principles.

Profession An occupation that involves professional training for individuals who adhere to ethical standards.

Professional A person who belongs to a profession.

REFERENCES

Ahrens Exercise Physiology. Home Page, [Online], http://www.ahrensep.com/

American Society of Exercise Physiologists. ASEP Accreditation Guidelines, [Online], http://www.asep.org/services/accreditation

American Society of Exercise Physiologists. Board Certified Exercise Physiologists, [Online], http://www.asep.org/people/certifiedEPs

American Society of Exercise Physiologists. Code of Ethics, [Online], http://www.asep.org/organization/ethics

American Society of Exercise Physiologists. ASEP Definition of Exercise Physiologists, [Online], http://www.asep.org/

American Society of Exercise Physiologists. ASEP Goals and Objectives, [Online], http://www.asep.org/general/goals

American Society of Exercise Physiologists. Home Page [Online], http://www.asep.org/

American Society of Exercise Physiologists. ASEP Vision Statement, [Online], http://www.asep.org/organization

Boone, T (2002) The psychocultural science of taking responsibility *Professionalization of Exercise Physiologyonline,* 5 [Online], http://faculty.css.edu/tboone2/asep/PsychoculturalSCIENCE.html

Boone, T (2007a) *Ethical standards and professional credentials in the practice of exercise physiology.* The Edwin Mellen Press, Lewiston, New York.

Boone, T (2007b) Power, politics, and the future *Professionalization of Exercise Physiologyonline,* 10 [Online], http://faculty.css.edu/tboone2/asep/PowerPOLITICSandFUTURE.html

Boone, T (2009) *The professionalization of exercise physiology: certification, accreditation, and standards of practice of the American Society of Exercise Physiologists (ASEP).* The Edwin Mellen Press, Lewiston, New York.

Boone, T (2010) Exercise science is a meaningless degree *Professionalization of Exercise Physiologyonline,* 13 [Online], http://faculty.css.edu/tboone2/asep/ExerciseScienceDegree.docx

Bruhn, JG (2001) Being good and doing good: the culture of professionalism in the health professions. *Health Care Manag (Frederick),* 19, 47-58.
[http://dx.doi.org/10.1097/00126450-200119040-00008] [PMID: 11411026]

Ciccolella, ME, Van Ness, JM & Boone, T (2008) A public at risk: personal fitness trainers without a standard of care *Professionalization of Exercise Physiology,* 11 [Online], http://faculty.css.edu/tboone2/asep/PublicAtRiskTrainers.html

Clinical Exercise Physiology Association. Home Page, [Online], http://www.acsm-cepa.org/i4a/pages/index.cfm?pageid=1

Etizioni, A (1969) *The semi-professions and their organizations.* The Free Press, New York, New York.

Greenwood, E (1957) Attributes of a profession. *Soc Work,* 3, 45-55.

Maxwell, JC (2003) *Thinking for a change.* Center Stree, New York, New York.

Rademacher, E & Pittsley, J (2001) Analysis and comparison of colleges and universities with degree titles of exercise physiology or related titles *Professionalization of Exercise Physiologyonline,* 4 [Online], http://faculty.css.edu/tboone2/asep/MinimalStandards.html

CHAPTER 15

Professionalization and Healthcare

Abstract: Exercise physiologists should focus on the professionalization of exercise physiology by supporting the American Society of Exercise Physiologists (ASEP), particularly in regards to their role in prescribing exercise medicine? Secondly, the non-academic community of non-doctorate exercise physiologists must provide a stronger voice for exercise physiology as a healthcare profession. It is important that exercise physiologists should focus on healthcare employment, and they must be taught the exercise physiologists' code of ethics and professional standards. For the profession of exercise physiology to become equal to physical therapy and other healthcare professions, members must help ensure that professionalism is at the core of the academic curriculum. The exercise prescription must be properly prescribed with specificity to promote positive outcomes and reduce complications. Age-related changes in human organ subsystems can be improved by regular exercise, but only if it is safely administered by ASEP Board Certified Exercise Physiologists.

Keywords: Credibility, Dishonesty, Entrepreneurs, Exercise science, Healthcare, Health promotion, Legal liability, Professionalization, Professional values.

INTRODUCTION

It is obvious that research is important for all the obvious reasons. This includes published papers with a molecular and cellular focus on exercise training as well as research that helps to explain the effects of regular exercise in the etiology and treatment of diseases (Baldwin 2000). So, where do exercise physiologists go from here? It is the author's perspective that research must continue for all the obvious reasons. However, exercise physiologists should also focus on the professionalization of exercise physiology, particularly in regards to their role in prescribing exercise medicine? Note that "exercise is medicine" and, therefore, exercise medicine can improve health and well-being. In fact, it is tragic that so little has been done by exercise physiologists to emphasize the healthcare factor of the profession.

At this point in time, physical inactivity is a much more pressing issue than the athlete's physical performance (Box **1**). Not only is it a critical healthcare need to find a way to get society to exercise, it is absolutely critical that Board Certified Exercise Physiologists are the key exercise-healthcare providers in the 21st century. The scientific evidence is clear that exercise can help prevent (and treat as well) chronic diseases and disabilities (such as diabetes, high blood pressure, colon and breast cancer, osteoporosis, depression, and dementia) (Boone 2016).

Box 1. Exercise medicine.

Exercise physiologists have known for decades that exercise is medicine. The scientific evidence is clear. Regular exercise helps to prevent chronic disease and premature death. Exercise physiologists are "the" healthcare providers of exercise medicine.

So, given this information, what are academic exercise physiologists waiting for? Why are they so slow in supporting ASEP as their professional organization? Exercise physiologists who are not members of a professional infrastructure will not be able to compete with healthcare professionals who are supporting their own professions. This is why exercise physiologists of the 21st century must develop and promote a strong and diverse knowledge base in both the science of exercise medicine and the professionalism of exercise physiology.

Type 2 diabetes patients can either be cured or markedly improved by engaging in regular exercise and a proper diet. But, it is important that with an increase in emphasis on exercise medicine the right healthcare professionals are involved. The ASEP Board Certified Exercise Physiologists are the right healthcare professionals to get clients and patients more active (Boone 2016). For this reason, the ASEP leaders are doing everything they can to ensure that Board Certified Exercise Physiologists are engaged in promoting professionalism.

Two critically important issues need to be addressed. Firstly, academic exercise physiologists need to promote the professional development of exercise physiologists by supporting the American Society of Exercise Physiologists.

Secondly, the non-academic community of non-doctorate exercise physiologists must provide a stronger voice for exercise physiology as a healthcare profession. As it stands, the lack of full support of the ASEP organization is the primary failing of the academic exercise physiologists in the United States.

As a parallel concept, historically, it was believed that drinking water during athletic training and performance was a sign of weakness (Stone *et al.* 2004). Now everyone knows that there are important reasons to drink water during training and/or a sporting event. Coaches are much better leaders today because they have learned to think outside the box. The group with the right ideas is the one with the power. Clearly, there are exercise physiologists without a plan and, consequently, they have no power. Moreover, they are their own worst enemy when it comes to not writing about professionalism. If their existence is only for publishing research papers, one has to wonder why they fail to realize the value in building their own profession of exercise physiology. It is obvious that exercise physiology meets the definition of a *profession*. The question is whether exercise physiologists know it or know what to do with the information.

Exercise physiologists provide society with an essential service (*i.e.,* exercise medicine), which is scientifically designed to benefit the recipients of that service (Box **2**). The professional service requires a mastery of a body of knowledge that is defined by the ASEP scope of practice and is regulated by the ASEP code of ethics (Begun & Lippincott 1993); all of which has been address dozens of times in professionalism articles published in the ASEP Professionalization of Exercise Physiology-online electronic journal (Boone 2004).

Box 2. Exercise physiology = exercise medicine.

Exercise physiologists have an important responsibility to be the glue that keeps exercise medicine at the very center of its professional development. After all, as John Maynard Keynes said, "The difficulty is not so much in developing new ideas as in escaping from the old ones."

The first step on the journey to success is no doubt the hardest. Whether it is three 50-minute periods of low to moderate exercise each week or the creation of professional development course in the exercise physiology curriculum, it is imperative that the first-step is taken. This is true for exercise medicine, and it is true for the commitment to professionalism in exercise physiology.

This thinking is not complicated by any means, yet so many academic exercise physiologists appear controlled by groupthink. It is against this backdrop that the ASEP leaders share their beliefs for nothing less than the exercise physiologist's recognition as a healthcare professional. They believe that healthcare in the future will increasingly focus on promoting health and wellness instead of just treating illnesses (Ryan 1998).

ASEP Board Certified Exercise Physiologists are expected to be key players in their own community-based healthcare practices, especially designed for health promotion and disease prevention. Their professional expertise is applicable to health promotion that includes cardiovascular assessments to assist clients in developing health promotion paths and in tracking their performance. It also means that the exercise physiologist of the future will work with clients who have spirituality concerns (Boone 2010). It is part of the striving towards discovering the purpose of exercise physiology as a scientific-based healthcare profession.

Healthcare is a trillion-dollar industry, representing about 14% of the U.S. gross domestic product (Woerner 1998). Healthcare is at the center of the ASEP's work. Now is the time to position Board Certified Exercise Physiologists as a powerful and essential force in healthcare. Hence, it is important that exercise physiologists focus on healthcare employment. After all, the benefits of regular exercise in the prevention of chronic disease and lowering of mortality rates are scientifically documented.

The changing landscape of healthcare is directly related to an increased need and demand for professional accountability. This is why the exercise physiologist's professional practice is important in maintaining competency that will assure the public is safe. The ASEP leaders believe that Board Certification is critical to facilitating consensus, increasing communication, and developing political awareness. This is why professional values such as ethics, integrity, altruism, and autonomy must be learned and reinforced in educational and practice settings.

Students do not automatically know or understand these points. They do not enter college understanding professionalism (Boone 2001), moral principles that include, but are not limited to, beneficence, nonmaleficence, veracity, and confidentiality, and the importance of a profession-specific code of ethics. They must be taught the exercise physiologist's code of ethics and professional practice standards. Otherwise, students (like most individuals) will follow the behavior of others (*e.g.,* their teachers) and do so automatically without thinking. This seems to be the case with regards to sports and performance enhancing supplements and drugs (Boone 2009a).

Change is a Certainty

For the profession of exercise physiology to become equal to physical therapy or other healthcare professions, members must help to ensure that professionalism is at the core of the academic curriculum. Academic exercise physiologists must be protected against certain mean spirited individuals, especially the negative aspects of groupthink, politics, and greed. Non-tenured exercise physiologists must be aware of the risk to their academic status, especially in the evaluation of how to respond to threats to their own academic position (Box **3**). The ASEP leaders must continue to establish policies and, where appropriate, institute measures designed to protect faculty members who support and promote the ASEP vision.

Box 3. Change is a function of time.

As is true with most organizations, change, development, and recognition are always a function of time. Patience is not wasted on doing the right thing for the right reason. Also, it is extremely important to never give up, never take a back seat, and never take "no" for an answer.

Exercise physiologists are the sole architect of their profession. Those who get this point understand there can be little doubt that exercise physiologists need their own professional organization. This shift from a generic organization to a professional one will continue to influence academic exercise physiologists. One reason is the growing awareness that the education of exercise physiologists as healthcare professionals brings with it liability issues concerning the protection of the public from incompetent college graduates and/or faculty (Brent 1007).

Academic exercise physiologists are not exempt from legal liability issues that result from avoidable malpractice due, in part, to defective instruction and/or the lack of a shared support and promotion of professionalism. This is not to argue that professionalism does not exist among exercise physiologists or that the college teachers are not qualified to teach. The truth is most academic exercise physiologists are good people and are well-educated with good intentions. But, unfortunately, many of them either do not believe they have control over exercise physiology or they do not see how their influence can be responsible for change and success.

It is the ASEP leaders' belief that non-doctorate exercise physiologists of the 21st century will work in an environment in which they will help create a better healthcare system. As healthcare entrepreneurs, they will be prepared as scholars and practitioners, and they will be much more likely to attract success than failure (Box **4**). They will also have the intellectual training and academic rigor of an accredited program to ask questions, think critically, and synthesize both practical and scientific information.

Box 4. Why wait if it is right.

Martin Luther King, Jr. said that, "The time is always right to do what is right."

Moreover, given their increased hands-on laboratory experiences that are frequently associated with knowledge acquisition and problem-solving, they will be better prepared as active learners. The ASEP rethinking of undergraduate exercise physiology will help promote new academic courses that will encourage career opportunities. There will be courses on anatomy, business, marketing, entrepreneurship, and spirituality as well as a greater diversity and depth of other exercise physiology mind-body courses. Students will graduate with a greater sense of how to move into entrepreneurial roles, thus enabling them to have more control over their career and future finances as well as a much greater impact on consumer healthcare (and athletic) outcomes.

Past, Present, and the Future of Exercise Physiology

The population 65 years of age and older increased from 35 million in 2000 to 40 million in 2010. By 2020, individuals 65 and older is expected to increase to 55 million (Administration on Aging 2007). The musculoskeletal, physiologic, neurologic, and psychological changes in older adults are increasingly complex. Interestingly, many of the age-related changes in older clients and patients can be managed by regular exercise (*i.e.,* exercise medicine). But, given the condition of the individuals, the exercise prescription must be properly prescribed with specificity to promote positive outcomes and reduce complications. Age-related changes in human organ subsystems can be helped by regular exercise, but only if it is safely administered. After all, the scientific link is indisputable, given the linear relationship between regular exercise and health and wellness.

Functional capacity is an excellent objective quantification of a person's exercise tolerance. Research by Spin and colleagues (Spin *et al.* 2002) suggests that for an increase in every 1 metabolic equivalent (*i.e.,* 1 MET; a unit used to estimate the amount of oxygen used by the body at rest and during physical activity) due to training, there is a reduction in annual mortality of 11%. This means that adults with have high blood pressure, decreased cardiac output, ventricular arrhythmias, and/or who may be taking β-blockers with chronic heart failure and ischemic heart disease will benefit from being tested by an ASEP Board Certified Exercise Physiologist.

Under no circumstances is the personal trainer or fitness instructor qualified to administer a graded exercise test that includes a comprehensive cardiovascular and metabolic assessment. Personal trainers have little to no actual academic training in age-related changes of the respiratory system, such as a loss of elastic recoil of the lung, decreased strength of the respiratory muscles, and decreased compliance of the chest wall. They are not aware that the changes lead to a decrease in tidal volume along with an increase in frequency of breaths that increase the work of breathing (Talley & Talley 2009). Also, they are aware of the changes that influence the cardiovascular system and tissue extraction.

The future of exercise physiology resides in healthcare (Box **5**). This does not diminish its past or its future role in sports, athletics, and/or fitness. However, without an entrepreneurial healthcare component to the exercise physiologist's career options, the students who major in exercise physiology will suffer the same job-related problems if not age-related academic problems as students of exercise science find themselves. This point was highlighted in 2006 by Roberta Rikli who said, "...together with a lack of a common name and common purpose has raised concern about the field's identity and importance in higher education...."

Box 5. Think about it.

In California alone, in 2005, the medical costs attributed to inactivity were estimated at $29 billion. This figure increases each year, as more people become inactive, given that sedentary lifestyles increase all causes of mortality.

The fact is that many professionals, including much of society, do not have any idea what career opportunities are available to exercise science graduates. Clearly, the lack of a professional philosophy and culture to sustain and clarify its role in the public sector, exercise science and the thousands of students majoring in related degree programs lack the professional infrastructure and credibility important to generate a financial income sufficient to raise a family. It is not that physical education, exercise science, or kinesiology students and their faculty do not understand the power of physical activity. Rather, understanding the power of exercise must come from an integrated and comprehensive academic program that is constantly being transformed by a healthcare focus.

The "Report" by James B. Conant (1963) was wrong in its assessment of physical education not having a sufficient scientific base to justify it as an academic field. Yet, given the nature of academia, the activity-oriented dimensions of physical education, and the lack of a heavy-based scientific curriculum, hardly anyone jumped up and disagreed. Instead, academic departments throughout the United States changed their names to exercise science. For whatever reason, they thought the word "science" was sufficient to keep the departments from being eliminated. As it turned out, the departments survived but not without issues that continue to compromise the lives of thousands of students. The problem is there was then, and there still is now a lack of visionary leaders (Box **6**).

Box 6. Every profession needs visionary leaders.

Leadership is always a function of risking failure, which is simply part of the process of changing, growing, and thinking differently (however unpopular the thoughts may be). So, get used to being uncomfortable. Being a leader is about the right attitude, staying strong, disciplined, and determined. It is also about the commitment to finding solutions to our problems.

In retrospect, from the beginning, it was not a good idea that every science-related course (*e.g.,* sports biomechanics, sports nutrition, sports psychology, and so forth) within physical education should become subdisciplines. Even today, there is relatively little to no collaboration across these fields of study. Much like the big bang theory, every department (chair and faculty) and every subdiscipline went in multiple different directions. Worse yet, given the lack of success, except to a large degree, exercise physiology, they are still moving apart from each other.

Only the profession of exercise physiology is for the most part a recognized composite of the course work from each of the original subdisciplines (Ellis 1998; Wilmore 1998).

Leadership and a Unified Front

Most college teachers understand that administrators are always looking for ways to contain costs even if it means getting rid of an academic program to reduce the size of the faculty and overhead expenses. The ASEP leaders understand this basic instinct to downsize, that is, as long as it is fair and driven by integrity. In many ways, they get what many of their colleagues do not get. They get the need to come together, to see the big-picture, and to think in a forward looking manner. This thinking is no doubt surprising since so many exercise physiologists remain non-ASEP members. It is as though they actually cannot see beyond their present research emphasis.

"Hello, wake up American" is a popular expression that is used to get people's attention. Similarly, it isn't hard to find an ASEP leader saying, "Hello, wake up exercise physiologists." By accepting personal responsibility for professionalism in exercise physiology, they will avoid the demise of exercise physiology along with the related academic degrees, such as has happened with UCLA (Scanlan 1998). It was once the Department of Kinesiology that had exercise physiologists as faculty members. Then, the name changed to the Department of Physiological Science. Today, it is the Department of Integrative Biology and Physiology. The majority of the 21 or so faculty members are not exercise physiologists.

Exercise physiology no longer exists at UCLA. The following statement was taken from the undergraduate Internet webpage of the department (UCLA

Department of Integrative Biology and Physiology 2010): "Physiological Science provides a rich background that covers cellular through whole organism physiology, and is appropriate for a variety of professions. Many of our students consider themselves Pre-Med, which means that they are satisfying requirements for entering Medical School upon graduation, or in the near future. Others seek rewarding careers in research, teaching, physical therapy, nursing, optometry and pharmacy, just to name a few options." This means that the physiological science major is as meaningless as is the exercise science major. Why? Because, now, the students must seek yet another academic degree to find employment in the public sector.

Once again, life repeats itself. If only exercise physiologists would unite and stop the fragmentation within exercise physiology, they would likely find a way to gain universal recognition and stability as an academic department. Doing so would help inform the public sector and other healthcare professions that exercise physiology is recognized as "the" authority in the assessment and prescription of exercise medicine. It is the heart of exercise physiology, not sports or strength training.

However, the exercise physiology community has resisted attempts to help it think differently. What is missing is the academic leadership outside of the ASEP organization to share in the work towards a unified mission to connect with and promote the ASEP vision. Frankly, that just does not make sense. The power of many isn't a joke. Every exercise physiologist has an equal responsibility in caring for and nurturing the profession (Box 7). Whether it is a professor talking about ASEP or the networking that takes place among many students, faculty, and their friends and colleagues, it is about the passion to convince colleagues of the value of coming together.

Box 7. The essential first step is to support ASEP.

If exercise physiologists fail to take care of the profession of exercise physiology, who do you think will step up to the plate and take control of it? The answer is not complicated, and it is actually a rather dangerous way to think. Yet, every day exercise physiologists fail to speak up and take action, the likelihood of another organization taking control increases. An essential first step is to get the members to be more active in ASEP.

John Maynard Keynes (Boone 2009b) said, "The hardest thing is not to get people to accept new ideas; it is to get them to forget old ones." That is the vital sign, isn't it? During the 20th century, the focus was on performing good research. Now, in the 21st century, the focus should be on professionalism and professional development. Exercise physiologists are living on the cusp of the transition between the two ages. The view of the ASEP leaders is different from the sports medicine view. They have opened a fabulous new window of opportunity to take control of exercise physiology.

But, first, to understand that exercise physiologists are responsible for nurturing professionalism, they must start paying closer attention to ASEP and its action points (Box **8**). Thus, it is important to that the objective of the study of exercise physiology is not just about how the body functions at rest and during exercise conditions. Knowing the physiological mechanisms of the adaptation process is required, but there must also be an integrated understanding of professionalism as well.

Box 8. The duty to share the ASEP vision.

There is no better indicator of a person's thinking than his/her action or the lack of it. Why exercise physiologists continue to ignore what is obvious is very much like dealing with a client who is living a sedentary lifestyle but will not take a brisk walk. Shouldn't they be advised on the importance of being more active in ASEP to increase membership and support? Academic exercise physiologists have a duty to share the ASEP vision with their students and make sure they understand the importance of professionalism in exercise physiology.

Are exercise physiologists ready for a change? Are the college teachers willing to become the master architect of a better future for all exercise physiologists? Change is always difficult. It means letting go of status quo and taking on a new perspective. Exercise physiologists must be willing to leave some things behind them so they can embrace a new future. Think for a moment about the following questions:

1. Will exercise physiologists become the architect of change within their own profession?
2. Will they become advocates of their professional organization?
3. Will they accept themselves as healthcare professionals, acknowledge their

problems, and rely on their own intellect and skills?

4. Will they accept that exercise science is a broken record and that sports medicine has no business acting like an exercise physiology organization?

Final Thoughts

The leaders of exercise physiology must develop strategies to unify the profession to help support a better healthcare team. The existing system does not make sense. Students should be required to take business and management courses during their undergraduate formative years of study. Graduate education must be more than statistics and research. It must be designed to teach students how to work in teams during their academic course work, particularly during the hands-own laboratory experiences.

Students must be taught how to develop business plans to maximize their career in healthcare and opportunities as entrepreneurs. Future exercise physiology leaders must go beyond the need to develop expertise in research to that of understanding a broad range of regulatory measures contributing to a new vision and dream for a professional healthcare practice (Box **9**). The potential for a very positive and successful transition is increased with the ASEP university-based accreditation, mentors, and emphasis on undergraduate scholarship and relevant work towards achieving professional development.

Box 9. Illusion or reality.

The student looks upon the college as a medium of pursuing dreams. -- Buzzle.com/ (2010)

The goal of the ASEP organization is to facilitate optimal client health through primary, secondary, and tertiary prevention interventions. Exercise medicine fits well with the "big picture" holistic concept of optimizing a dynamic and stable interrelationship of mind, spirit, and body of all clients. The good news is that a lot of work has already been done. Now, today, exercise physiologists can change their beliefs, they can teach anatomy and provide hands-on anatomy laboratory opportunities (Box **10**), and they can "walk the walk, talk the talk" to demonstrate their responsibility in defining the 21st century future of exercise physiology as a healthcare profession.

Box 10. Will exercise physiologists meet the challenge?

The importance of studying anatomy (as a critical piece of the students' education), the need to use research findings in the ASEP practice, the willingness to change, and the need for professionalism in exercise physiology are all important for survival. The question is this: Will exercise physiologists meet the challenge? The ASEP leaders think so.

GLOSSORY

Credibility	The quality of being trustworthy and believable.
Dishonesty	The display of behavior that is deceitful and not worthy of trusting.
Entrepreneur	A person who organizes and manages a business.
Healthcare	The prevention, treatment, or restoration of the health of the body and mind.
Legal liability	Legal responsibility for one's acts or omissions.
Values	The judgment of what is important in life and work.

REFERENCES

Administration on Aging, US Department of Health and Human Services, A profile of older Americans. [Online], http://www.agingcarefl.org/aging/AOA-2007profile.pdf

Baldwin, KM (2000) Research in the exercise sciences: where do we go from here? *Journal of Applied Physiology,* 88, 332-6.
[PMID: 10642398]

Begun, JW & Lippincott, RC (1993) *Strategic adaptation in the health professions.* Jossey-Bass, San Francisco, CA.

Boone, T (2001) *Professional development of exercise physiology.* The Edwin Mellen Press, Lewiston, New York.

Boone, T (2004) The impact factor: a critical review *Professionalization of Exercise Physiologyonline,* 7 [Online], http://faculty.css.edu/tboone2/asep/journalIMPACTfactor.html

Boone, T (2009a) *Basic issues in sports ethics: the many ways of cheating.* The Edwin Mellen Press, Lewiston, New York.

Boone, T (2009b) Leadership: encouraging the change process *Professionalization of Exercise Physiologyonline,* 12 [Online], http://faculty.css.edu/tboone2/asep/Leadership2009.pdf

Boone, T (2010) *Integrating spirituality and exercise physiology: toward a new understanding of health.* The

Edwin Mellen Press, Lewiston, New York.

Boone, T (2016) *ASEP's exercise medicine text for exercise physiologists.* Bentham Science Publishers, Beijing, China.
[http://dx.doi.org/10.2174/97816810832161160101]

Brent, J (1997) *Nurses and the law: a guide to principles and applications.* W. B. Saunders, Philadelphia, Pennsylvania.

Buzzle.com/ Purpose of college education. [Online], http://www.buzzle.com/articles/ purpose-of-colle-e-education.html

Conant, JB (1963) *The education of American teachers.* McGraw-Hill, New York, New York.

Ellis, MJ (1998) Disasters on the west coast: personal observations. *Quest,* 50, 116-20.
[http://dx.doi.org/10.1080/00336297.1998.10484269]

Rikli, RE (2006) Kinesiology – a "homeless" field: addressing organization and leadership needs. National Association for Kinesiology and Physical Education in Higher Education. *Quest,* 58, 288-309.
[http://dx.doi.org/10.1080/00336297.2006.10491884]

Ryan, S (1998) *Education and partnerships in the global community, Unpublished presentation at Health Care Resources.* HCR, Rochester, New York.

Scanlan, TK (1998) Thriving *versus* surviving. *Quest,* 50, 126-33.
[http://dx.doi.org/10.1080/00336297.1998.10484270]

Spin, JM, Prakash, M, Froelicher, VF, Partington, S, Marcus, R, Do, D & Myers, J (2002) The prognostic value of exercise testing in elderly men. *American Journal of Medicine,* 112, 453-9.
[http://dx.doi.org/10.1016/S0002-9343(02)01065-3] [PMID: 11959055]

Stone, MH, Sands, WA & Stone, ME (2004) The downfall of sports science in the United States. *National Strength and Conditioning Association,* 26, 72-5.
[http://dx.doi.org/10.1519/00126548-200404000-00014]

Talley, HC & Talley, CH (2009) AANA Journal course. Update for nurse anesthetists. Evaluation of older adults. *American Association of Nurse Anesthetists Journal,* 77, 451-60.
[PMID: 20108733]

UCLA Department of Integrative Biology and Physiology. Undergraduate program, [Online], http://www.physci.ucla.edu/undergraduate.php

Wilmore, JH (1998) Building strong academic programs for our future. *Quest,* 50, 103-7.
[http://dx.doi.org/10.1080/00336297.1998.10484266]

Woerner, L (1998) *Health care: whose business is it?.*

CHAPTER 16

The Future: Curriculum Change

Abstract: Is it realistic that academic exercise physiologists teach anatomy in the exercise physiology curriculum? If so, is it necessary that they studied anatomy in their doctorate program? If they did not study anatomy and/or dissect cadavers, is it reasonable to expect them to know anatomy? If it is not reasonable, then, should the exercise physiology doctorate curriculum change to better educate the students of the 21st century? After all, exercise physiologists are healthcare professionals and, therefore, they must have the opportunity to study and dissect cadavers in the same way that other healthcare professionals have. The power of anatomy in identifying the right and the wrong way to lift weights, to increase range of motion, and to develop the motor aspects of physical skills is testament to its importance. This requires exercise physiology educators to take seriously the learning of anatomy as a dynamic basis for solving health and athletic problems.

Keywords: Board certification, Career opportunities, Curriculum, Osteological, Specialist, Teachers.

INTRODUCTION

A colleague stated it is unrealistic to expect that academic exercise physiologists will teach anatomy. They are not interested in anatomy. They are interested in research and physiology. A student who heard the professor asked: "How can exercise physiologists simply avoid teaching anatomy?" "Knowledge of anatomy is critical to the practice of exercise physiology. Isn't anatomy a critical part of becoming a healthcare professional?" Another student asked, "Why is ECG and graded exercise testing more important than anatomy?" She felt that the comment by the faculty member did not make sense. They felt it was important to teach anatomy, and that the emphasis on anatomy in sports and healthcare should be equal to other subjects in the exercise physiology curriculum.

Tommy Boone

Updating and managing curriculum changes is never an easy process or otherwise more college teachers, chairs, and directors would be more inclined to review existing courses in lieu of new courses (Boone 2009). The purpose of this book is to help exercise physiologists recognize that there are critical issues in exercise physiology that need timely and purposeful consideration. Students who want to be exercise physiologists need the appropriate time and commitment to anatomy and the physiological inroads into understanding human movement (*i.e.,* regular exercise and/or athletics). It is the experience of most healthcare professionals that anatomy is critical to the students' education and career opportunities.

The Re-Examination Process

The review process offers the opportunity to examine what is taught and to ask questions whether change is necessary. What is critical to understand is that the curriculum must allow for accomplishing the desired outcomes that allow for the graduate to perform as a professional. It also provides the impetus for changing the emphasis on certain courses in consideration of what is believed more important (Boone 2007). The point is this: The curriculum should match up with the purpose of the degree itself, which raises the following questions:

1. What is the reason for the degree in exercise physiology?
2. Why does exercise physiology exists as an academic major?
3. Is it a technical degree?
4. Is it a research degree?
5. It is a clinical degree?
6. Is it a sports-oriented degree and, if so, which sport?
7. Is it an exercise instructor's degree?
8. Is it a personal trainer degree?
9. Is it a healthcare degree?
10. Is it a professional degree?

Shouldn't the design of the curriculum be driven by the definition of exercise physiology? If so, what is the professional definition of exercise physiology? Who is an exercise physiologist (Boone 2005)? The definition of exercise physiology by the American Society of Exercise Physiologists (ASEP 2016) bears repeating.

"Exercise Physiology is the identification of physiological mechanisms underlying physical activity, the comprehensive delivery of treatment services concerned with the analysis, improvement, and maintenance of health and fitness, rehabilitation of heart disease and other chronic diseases and/or disabilities, and the professional guidance and counsel of athletes and others interested in athletics, sports training, and human adaptability to acute and chronic exercise." Clearly, the exercise physiology academic major is a professional healthcare major.

Also, as previously described, the ASEP leaders (Boone 2001) defined the "Exercise Physiologist as a person who has an academic degree in exercise physiology, or who is certified by ASEP to practice exercise physiology [*via* the Exercise Physiologist Certified exam (EPC)], or who has a doctorate degree with an academic degree or emphasis in exercise physiology from an accredited college or university." Once again, it is clear that the graduate of an exercise science major is not an exercise physiologist unless he or she engages additional study and passes the ASEP Board Certification (EPC) exam. Although at present there are a number of ways in which a person can achieve the objective of earning the professional title, Exercise Physiologist, the ASEP intent is to move towards the adoption of only graduates from the academic exercise physiology major as having the right to call themselves exercise physiologists.

The whole process of curriculum review must be built upon a 21st century philosophy of exercise physiology (Boone 2014). The sports medicine approach is outdated, particularly since it has also failed to acknowledge the key role of anatomy in exercise physiology. It is the experience of the author that the presence of one of more exercise physiologists with training in cadaver dissection is beneficial not only in the important aspect of curricular review, but also in the subsequent agreement as to what should be taught. The purpose is to help facilitate the objective that anatomy is important and that the strengths of anatomy further define the credibility of the exercise physiology practice.

A detailed knowledge of anatomy forms the basis for much of the healthcare work that Board Certified Exercise Physiologists will do with patients and clients. The latter is especially the case common among athletes interested in specific muscular development. The power of anatomy is the identification of the right way to lift weights, to increase range of motion, and to develop the right motor skills. Not only are there educational and professional reasons to teach anatomy, there are also litigious reasons that support the exercise physiologists' need for anatomical knowledge (Box **1**).

Box 1. Think about…by comparison.

The mass media have recently reported unacceptable levels of morbidity and mortality based on physician incompetence (Gawande 1999); 51.3 ± 6.9 percent of the deaths from adverse events were caused by negligence (Brennan *et al.* 1991). It is very likely that some of these deaths can be directly attributed to anatomic incompetence related to its diminished role in medical education. This is supported by a recent survey that showed that less than one-third of residency program directors indicated that new residents were adequately prepared in anatomy (Cahill *et al.* 2000).

If exercise physiologists do not know the difference between the muscle arising in part from the clavicle and the full length of the sternum and the muscle that arises from the outer surfaces of ribs three through five or the functional significance (or difference) between the brachialis, biceps brachii, and brachioradialis, there are going to be mistakes made with clients and patients (Box **2**).

Box 2. The power of knowledge.

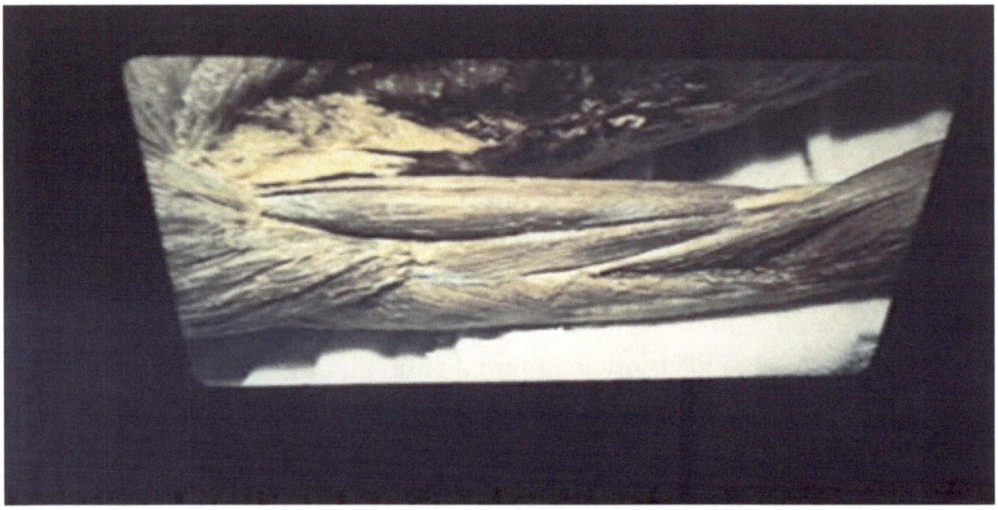

There is no question that a thorough knowledge and understanding of human anatomy underlies sound exercise physiology practice and, therefore, is an essential academic course in the students' undergraduate education. This thinking is so straight forward and so simple that it is next to impossible to imagine academic exercise physiologists who think otherwise. One must wonder, "Is it their education or the lack of it?"

With the decline in anatomical knowledge possessed by academic exercise physiologists, it is more than reasonable that the majority of the non-doctorate exercise physiologists cannot answer the following questions:

1. What is the anatomical connection between the pectineus and the psoas major and the muscle that arises from the anterior surface of the ileum?
2. Why are they innervated by the same nerve and insert into essentially the same osteological site?
3. What is the significance of the eight plantar flexors innervated by two nerves?
4. In what way are the nerves a product of the sciatic nerve?
5. Which muscle that inserts on the posterior surface of the calcaneus is the powerhouse of plantar flexors?
6. Why does sitting with a weight on the top of the knees during calf raises take an important plantar flexor out of action?
7. Which one of the two nerves to the "leg" innervates two of the eight plantar flexor muscles?

Final Thoughts

The answer to this state of affairs is to teach anatomy at the undergraduate level and the graduate levels (master's and doctorate). Also, it is important that the teachers of the anatomy course are exercise physiologists and not biologists or clinical specialists from other fields of study. This requires exercise physiology educators to take seriously the learning of anatomy as a dynamic basis for safely prescribing exercise medicine in healthcare settings and working with athletes.

Every student of exercise physiology should know the brachial plexus just as he or she is taught the steps of glycolysis, a dozen or so intricate biomechanical steps and formulae, research design and statistics, the reading of an ECG during a graded exercise test, and the cardiorespiratory calculations that are used to understand and describe an individual's physiology at rest and during exercise. Understandably, the barriers to teaching anatomy are significant. Aside from the shortage of qualified exercise physiologists to teach anatomy, there is the increased length of time required for the study of anatomy and when and if anatomy is taught by dissection. Nonetheless, anatomy education is essential part of the exercise physiology curriculum. It also helps to further the development of professionalism in exercise physiology.

With regards to the brachial plexus illustrated in Box **3**, the teacher of anatomy uses drawings and photographs from textbooks and slides from dissection during anatomy lectures to ask questions and discuss structure and function that should be part of the students' academic education in the exercise physiology major. This thinking is no different from the expectation that students can identify and understand the significance of a post-MI patient's PVCs on an ECG strip *vs.* a normal sinus rhythm minutes earlier during the progressive exercise test.

Box 3. Anatomy of the brachial plexus.

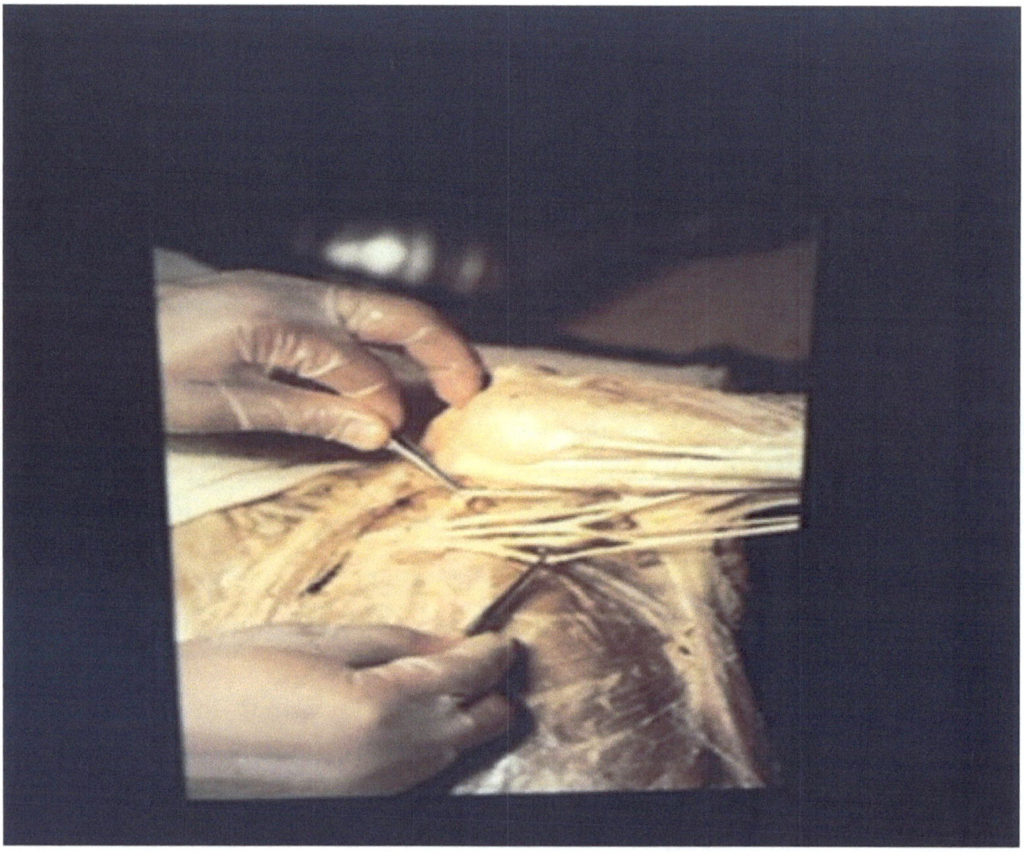

The teaching of anatomy must not be dismissed as obsolete (Older 2004).

GLOSSORY

Board certification	The process of examining and certifying the qualifications of an exercise physiologist or other professional by passing the "Exercise Physiologist Certified" (EPC) exam.
Career opportunities	Diverse and financially meaningful careers in exercise physiology as a Board Certified Exercise Physiologist.
Curriculum	The list of required academic courses necessary to comprehend the complexities of exercise physiology as a healthcare profession.
Osteological	The branch of anatomy that deals with the structure and function of bones.
Specialist	An exercise physiologist whose practice is limited to a particular branch of exercise physiology (such as research, athletic performance, or exercise medicine), especially one who is certified by the ASEP Board of Certification.
Teachers	Exercise physiologists whose interest is primarily teaching, such as in an academic institution.

REFERENCES

American Society of Exercise Physiologists. What is exercise physiology? [Online], http://www.asep.org/

Boone, T (2001) *Professional development of exercise physiology.* The Edwin Mellen Press, Lewiston, New York.

Boone, T (2005) *Exercise physiology: professional issues, organizational concerns, and ethical trends.* The Edwin Mellen Press, Lewiston, New York.

Boone, T (2007) *Ethical standards and professional credentials in the practice of exercise physiology.* The Edwin Mellen Press, Lewiston, New York.

Boone, T (2009) *The professionalization of exercise physiology: certification, accreditation, and standards of practice of the American Society of Exercise Physiologists (ASEP).* The Edwin Mellen Press, Lewiston, New York.

Boone, T (2014) *Introduction to exercise physiology.* Jones & Bartlett Publishing, Burlington, Massachusetts.

Brennan, TA, Leape, LL, Laird, NM, Hebert, L, Localio, AR, Lawthers, AG, Newhouse, JP, Weiler, PC & Hiatt, HH (1991) Incidence of adverse events and negligence in hospitalized patients. Results of the Harvard Medical Practice Study I. *New England Journal of Medicine,* 324, 370-6. [http://dx.doi.org/10.1056/NEJM199102073240604] [PMID: 1987460]

Cahill, DR, Leonard, RJ & Marks, SC, Jr (2000) A comment on recent teaching of human anatomy in the United States. *Surgical and Radiologic Anatomy,* 22, 69-71. [http://dx.doi.org/10.1007/s00276-000-0069-4] [PMID: 10959670]

Gawande, A (1999) When doctors make mistakes *The New Yorker,* February 1;40-55.

Older, J (2004) Anatomy: a must for teaching the next generation. *Surgeon,* 2, 79-90.

Epilogue: A Vision to Realize

INTRODUCTION

The right education contributes to professional and social change that is a critical step towards replacing present-day thinking with new ideas and possibilities. A major responsibility of the academic exercise physiologists is to help students realize their full potential as healthcare professionals. When the education of students includes anatomy (and, yes, cadaver dissection), exercise physiology will move closer to the reality of being a credible healthcare profession. Naturally, this is not going to happen overnight, but it must happen because anatomy teaching is an integral part of the students' professional education.

Hegelian scholar J. Glenn Gray (1984), in Re-Thinking American Education, makes a similar case when he said, "Only to the degree that we become educated, do we gain relationships of depth and intimacy to the encompassing world." "Becoming educated" is more than getting a college degree or even a doctorate degree. Without gaining the relationship of depth and intimacy to the exercise physiologists' world of scientific knowledge and hands-on experiences and the role of each in helping clients, one cannot help but feel loss and confused.

The education of exercise physiology students should be thoroughly thought out and implemented. It is about uncovering the entire complexity of the body, not just the physiology or even the biomechanics or nutritional needs of athletes. It is about the interconnection between anatomy, physiology, and the foundational sciences necessary to understand the vital connection between the mind and the body. Hence, it is by studying anatomy in the classroom and in the laboratory that the students of exercise physiology can be, as Greene (1988) said, "...empowered to think about what they are doing, to become mindful, to share meanings, to conceptualize...".

It is paramount that academic exercise physiologists see to it that their department produces exercise physiologists who are professionally competent and who have hands-on knowledge of anatomy. Indeed, college graduates need a new vision of the whole person, mind, muscles, and physiology. It is no longer sufficient for exercise physiologists to be anything less than what the ASEP vision entails.

To understand this point, the reader must grasp the exercise physiologists' vision (ASEP 2010). It is the most fundamental fact of why ASEP was founded in 1997. The vision is believed to be a much better idea whose time has come. Exercise physiology is not exercise science. Too many academic exercise physiologists go through their work every day clueless about what to do to empower the students and promote the profession of exercise physiology. Fortunately, ASEP exercise physiologists are defining these issues and problems whether it is in regards to health, fitness, rehabilitation, or athletics. They understand the vision of teaching anatomy generates hope and motivates the discouraged to stay the course.

That is why the ASEP vision explains what the ASEP leaders want (Box **1**), which is to be recognized as the leading professional organization of American scholars and practitioners in the study and application of exercise physiology to fitness, health promotion, rehabilitation, and sports training. ASEP is dedicated to unifying exercise physiologists in the United States by promoting and supporting the study, practice, teaching, research, and development of the profession of exercise physiology. Through proactive and creative leadership, the Society empowers its members to serve the public good by making an academically sound difference in the application of exercise physiology concepts and insights.

Box 1. A vision is magical and innovative.

The right vision can change everything about exercise physiology. It is the motivator to get exercise physiologists in the right frame of mind. It is the force that will impact and change the lives of thousands of students forever.

The essential point is this: The ASEP vision is a way of life to be lived. To be successful and appealing to exercise physiologists, it must not be viewed as impossible to attain. The ASEP leaders believe it is challenging and believable. Clearly, to make an academically sound difference in the application of exercise physiology concepts and insights, particularly in regards to exercise medicine, the exercise physiology educators must tackle the formidable problem of little to no anatomy instruction. One way of doing so is to make large-scale changes in the curricular. In short, this means doing what can be done with what one has until the process is well underway year after year. This is especially true during times of transition – such as when exercise physiologists are moving away from status quo and paying special attention to professionalism.

It is especially important to get the commitment of the academic professors who are directly responsible for implementing the change with their actions and words. It is they who will be responsible for conveying the visionary message that it is not possible to fully teach exercise physiology students without teaching anatomy and finding a balance among the exercise physiology courses and hands-on skills.

Also, an important point is that while computer programs and plastic models can be useful adjuncts, the primary focus should be on the use of cadavers. But, of course, understanding that the benefits of using cadavers in teaching and learning anatomy at the non-doctorate level will not happen overnight, the immediate concern is to ensure that the doctorate level exercise physiology students will have the opportunity to study anatomy (Box **2**) with the use of both prosections and cadavers in the exercise physiology curriculum.

Box 2. Dissection of some of the muscles of the anterior, lateral, and posterior leg.

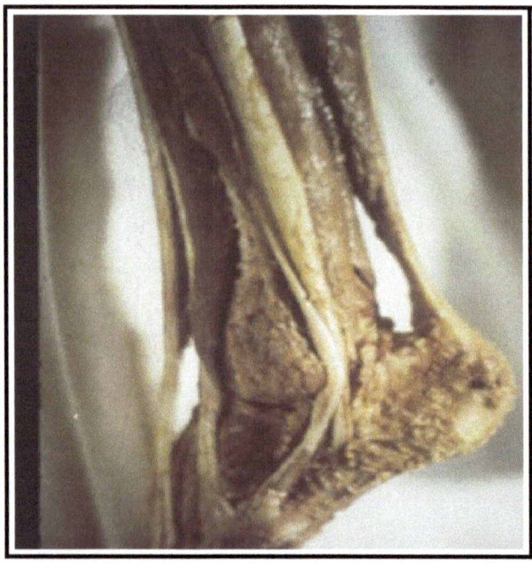

Note the five tendons from left to right.
1. **extensor digitorum longus** (originates from the anterior-lateral part of the leg)
2. **tibialis anterior** (originates in the upper two-thirds of the lateral surface of the tibia)
3. **peroneus brevis** (originates from the lower one-half of the lateral shaft of the fibula)
4. **peroneus longus** (originates from the head of fibula, upper one-half to two-thirds of the lateral side of the fibular)
5. **gastrocnemius** (originates from the lateral and medial condyles of the femur)

Question: Which one is a combination of two muscles?

Where possible both the undergraduate and the graduate students should be taught structural anatomy by lectures and complete dissection of the human body (Box **3**). Thus, to deal appropriately with this issue, there should be a full debate at every level of higher education to highlight areas of concern, to explore in depth the challenges, and to define a minimal core curriculum for the study of anatomy. The teaching of anatomy in exercise physiology must be valued, pursued, and experienced. Otherwise, it is more than reasonable to expect that the departments and institutions will be held liable for their training and teaching if they are shown to be insufficient for the safe practice of exercise medicine.

Box 3. The learning of anatomy is a visual and tactile experience.

Anatomical dissection is the systematic exploration of a preserved human cadaver by the sequential division of tissue layers and the liberation of certain structures by removal of the regional fat and connective tissue with the aim of supporting the learning of gross anatomy by visual and tactile experience.

-- Andreas Winkelmann (2006)

REFERENCES

American Society of Exercise Physiologists. *ASEP Vision.* Available from: http:// www.asep.org/vision

Gray, JG (1984) *Re-thinking American education a philosophy of teaching and learning* Wesleyan University Press, Connecticut, Massachusetts.

Greene, M (1988) *The dialectic of freedom.* Teachers College Press, New York, New York.

Winkelmann, A (2007) Anatomical dissection as a teaching method in medical school: a review of the evidence. *Med Educ,* 41, 15-22.
[http://dx.doi.org/10.1111/j.1365-2929.2006.02625.x] [PMID: 17209888]

SUBJECT INDEX

A

B

C

Tommy Boone

D

E

F

G

H

I

K

U

V

W

www.ingramcontent.com/pod-product-compliance
Lightning Source LLC
LaVergne TN
LVHW070935210926
848482LV00003B/246
* 9 7 8 1 6 8 1 0 8 4 7 0 1 *